Managing
Morning Sickness

A Survival Guide for
Pregnant Women

D1298729

Miriam Erick, R.D., M.S.

Bull Publishing Company
P.O. Box 1377
Boulder, CO 80306
Phone (800) 676-2855   Fax (303) 545-6354

ISBN 0-923521-82-8

Distributed to the trade by:
Publishers Group West
1700 Fourth Street
Berkeley, CA 94710

Publisher: James Bull
Developmental Editor: Erin Mulligan
Cover Design: Lightbourne
Interior Design: Linda Robertson
Composition: Publication Services, Inc.

This book is meant to educate, but should not be used as a substitute for professional
medical advice or care. The reader should consult her healthcare provider concerning
her individal pregnancy and medical condition and her pediatrician regarding her
baby. The author has done her best to ensure that the information presented here is
accurate up to the time of publication. However, as research and development are
ongoing, it is possible that new findings may supersede some of the information in
this edition.

Library of Congress Cataloging-in-Publication Data

Erick, Miriam.
  Managing morning sickness : a survival guide for pregnant women / by
Miriam Erick.— [Rev. ed.]
     p. cm.
  Rev. ed. of: No more morning sickness. New York : Plume, 1993.
  Includes bibliographical references and index.
  ISBN 0-923521-82-8
  1. Morning sickness—Prevention. I. Erick, Miriam. No more morning
sickness. II. Title.

  RG579.E73 2004
  618.2'4—dc22

2004005893

This book is dedicated to Agnes Hovi—
for all the wonderful lessons you taught me.
Kiitos!

Contents

Foreword

Nausea and vomiting of pregnancy (NVP) affects an estimated 80 percent of pregnant women. As such it is the most common medical condition in pregnancy. Sadly though, it is also the most ignored and neglected condition, leaving millions of women to suffer unnecessarily. Since we initiated the Motherisk NVP line in 1996, we have become painfully aware how much misinformation women deal with.

Ms. Erick should be congratulated for producing this fountain of information and personal stories. The book's strengths lie in the plethora of information about the condition, including its emotional, social, and historical aspects. There are numerous tips and suggestions for dietary solutions and remedies to alleviate NVP. Since it was not written as a "medical" book, readers may still need to research more information about the safety of some of the medications mentioned, as well as, possibly, the scientific evidence for some of the information. More information can be found in numerous other places, including on our own Web site (www.motherisk.org).

This volume is an important step in ensuring that women and their unborn babies are not orphaned from the benefit of advances in medicine.

Gideon Koren MD, FRCPC
Director and Senior Scientist, Motherisk Program
Professor of Pediatrics, Pharmacology, Pharmacy, Medicine.
  and Medical Genetics at the University of Toronto
Ivey Chair in Molecular Toxicology,
    University of Western Ontario

Acknowledgments

There are countless wonderful people who made this work a reality, to whom I am most indebted.

Thanks go to Jim Bull of Bull Publishing for producing this baby in about 9 months; to editor Erin Mulligan for keeping me on track and for her fabulous insight into organizing a book that was becoming more pregnant with every late-breaking medical report; to copy editor Alysia Cooley at Publication Services for her careful attention to detail throughout this book's gestation; and to Jan Fisher at Publication Services for the steady encouragement as the fatigue factor of the third trimester settled in!

I want to thank my witty and wonderful wordsmith friends—Kathleen Winkler, Kay Coleman, Tim Champion, David Priest, Elena Fechner, and Jack Brady—for sharing word power.

My colleagues in the Department of Nutrition and Food Services at Brigham and Women's Hospital—Kathy McManus, Karen Purdy-Reilly, Patsy Gleason-Clayton, Deirdre Ellard, Jen Evans, Marijane Staniec, Tricia DeGroot, Anar Shah, Julie

Redfern, and Caitlin Hosmer—deserve special thanks for their incredible friendship and support. I also want to thank all the great nurses with whom I work, especially those in obstetrics, neurology, surgery, and orthopedics.

All of these people were indispensable in providing stress reduction, computer-crash damage control, and good, old-fashioned laughs: Anastasia Michalowski, Martha Hunter, Carrie Kourmelis, Pastor Meg Hess, Sandy Sheiber, Ellyn Baltz, Tanya and David von Zurmuehlen, the O'Donnells and the Parklake Crew, Karen Shea, Jeanne Hamilton, Kay George, Linda Wilman, Mireille Stanbro, Anne Geuss, Jim Roche, Brian McDermott, Dan Hanna, Paul (my PC nerd), Daniel Kamman, Dick Doherty, Malcolm Johnson, Susan Sherman, and Tim O'Leary.

I am thankful for the privilege I have had to work beside some wonderful doctors at Brigham and Women's Hospital: Robert Barbieri (Chairman of the Department of Obstetrics and Gynecology), Louise Wilkins-Haug, Janis Fox, Mari-Kim Bunnell, David Acker, Nawal Nour, and dozens of others. I am also glad to have had the opportunity to work with fabulous colleagues at Massachusetts General Hospital, especially Fredric Frigoletto, Jr. and Jeff Ecker, and at Boston Medical Center, specifically Linda Heffner and Aviva Lee-Paritz.

I owe thanks to the following people for sharing their research and insights into this subject: Jeffrey Greenspoon, M.D. at UCLA; Leroy Heinrichs, M.D. at Stanford University; Dastur Fastad, Ph.D., Department of Psychology, Western Washington University; Teo Postolache, Ph.D. at the University of Maryland at Baltimore; Anthony R. Scialli, M.D. at Georgetown University; and Shari Munch, Ph.D., L.S.W. at Rutgers University.

Many thanks go to all my family for all their support—especially my nephews Chase, Andrew, Timmy, and Leif—and to my almost-sister and best pal, Sherri Hayes, at the University of Miami and her family for years of rest and relaxation and incredible friendship.

And lastly, a big thank you goes out to each of the countless morning-sick women who've tolerated extensive and exhaustive interviews so I could get the inside scoop.

Introduction

Ok. You're pregnant (drum roll please)—you are going to have a baby! Chances are you've thought about this on and off for a while—maybe you've even been through a round of fertility treatments and you thought the hard stuff was over. Or maybe you thought the tough part was deciding when to stop birth control because of your career and financial planning issues. Maybe your doctor told you the news or maybe you just turned green day one and there was no need for the rabbit test!

The events preceding every pregnancy are unique, but once that horrible nausea hits—the great nasty common denominator— you have lots of company on every corner of the planet. The occasional episode of vomiting you figured went with the territory may now be an everyday activity that's getting old fast. I'm guessing that you picked up this book because you are miserable and this pregnancy business just isn't what you imagined at all! Your productivity at work is falling, your social calendar is laced with cancellations, and the smallest household chore is almost as daunting as climbing Mt. Everest. You look like you've been hit by a bus—so much for all those glorious visions and expectations of "when I get pregnant it will be so much fun!"

There is no way to predict whether your morning sickness course will be a nuisance for a few weeks or you are headed for the "tough stuff." What you will learn from this book is how changing your diet can help—even if it means eating junk food for a few days or even a few weeks. You'll learn why you've developed the "radar nose of pregnancy" and why men can't detect their own "dog breath." You'll find lists of food therapies. You'll read a few medical case reports of really bad morning sickness to let you know you are definitely not alone, and it could be even worse! You will find Internet resources and information about medications and alternative therapies. You'll understand why it's easier to have a broken leg than to have invisible but chronic nausea that no one seems to be able to understand or treat successfully. You'll see how much more research the medical community needs to conduct to figure out the hormonal chaos you're going through. You'll read historical facts about morning sickness care from a hundred years ago and wonder how women survived!

Believe me I know exactly what you are going through— because I take care of women *just like you* every day of the year. I've spent the last year hunting down all the newest knowledge nuggets to help make your pregnancy less miserable. This book is *not* a substitute for medical care, but it may help your doctor as much as it will help you. Hopefully, this book will help you get through the toughest crises and, once you do, it will guide you through the steps you need to maintain healthy and optimal nutrition, because that is your (and your baby's) ticket to good health.

All the best!
Miriam

About the Author

Miriam Erick, known to her patients as the "morning sickness maven," has studied morning sickness, nausea and vomiting, and hyperemesis gravidarum for most of her career. She authored the classic primer, *No More Morning Sickness: A Survival Guide for Pregnant Women* (1993), which was awarded the Pyramid Award for distinguished medical communication by the New England chapter of the American Medical Writers Association in 1994.

Her serious cartoon book *Take Two Crackers and Call Me in the Morning! A Real-Life Guide for Surviving Morning Sickness* was produced in 1995 and subsequently translated into Spanish, making it the first morning-sickness resource for Spanish-speaking women. Miriam made her film debut in the 1995 video *Morning Sickness: All Day and All Night,* by Lemonaid Films, co-starring with many of her actual patients.

Nominated by nutrition colleagues, she shared the American Dietetic Association Foundation Ross Award for Women's Health in 1996 for her morning sickness advocacy work. Her common-sense approach, which takes into account the enhanced olfaction and sensory acuity of pregnancy and focuses on the benefits of an organoleptic diet, has improved the well-being of many thousands of pregnant women worldwide.

An avid medical writer and accomplished public speaker, Miriam is an educational affiliate of the American College of Obstetrics and Gynecology. She is also a member of the American Dietetics Association, the practice groups of Dietitians in Nutrition Support and Women's Health and Reproductive Nutrition, and the Massachusetts Dietetic Association. In addition she serves on the editorial board of *SHAPE* magazine.

Miriam is a certified diabetes educator and a senior clinical Registered Dietitian at Brigham and Women's Hospital in Boston, Massachusetts, where she also established the Morning Sickness Nutrition Clinic for the Departments of Nutrition and Obstetrics. She lives in the metropolitan Boston area with two inspiring cats, Razor Blades and Ms. Lucy.

Chapter 1

What Is Morning Sickness, Anyway?

AMY

Amy had an uneventful second pregnancy, and, based on what she told me, she deserved it! Two years earlier, at age 22, she'd become pregnant for the first time. At that time she lived with her husband in a town on the Rhode Island coast. Her nausea and vomiting started at the beginning of August, in the second month of her pregnancy.

Thus began her encampment in the master bedroom, near an overworked air conditioner. Living on iced tea, Amy could tolerate cold fruit salad only when she was feeling "better." That particular summer was unbearably hot and humid. She described the foods she could stomach as "cold"; she even ate cold bread. She found it easier to breathe if the air was also extremely cold. Hot, humid air made her breathless and instantly nauseated. She would wrap herself up in a winter blanket and stay in her air-conditioned bedroom for days on end.

Amy was 5 feet, 4 inches tall; she started her pregnancy a bit overweight at 150 pounds. By November, her fifth month, her weight was down to 147 pounds. At this point in her pregnancy, she should have weighed 6 to 10 pounds more than her prepregnancy weight, but she had a calculated gross deficit of 9 to 13 pounds, based on her expected weight. It was odd that no one seemed to notice she was melting away pound by pound. (Compare Amy's weight to the generic weight grid in Appendix A.)

When the heater was turned on for the first time in November, Amy reacted poorly to the smell. She described it as "roasted dust." She had not been well enough to do the usual fall cleaning, which included vacuuming the radiators. When the scorched dust smell abated, her gastrointestinal equilibrium returned.

In January, at her seventh month, she had strong cravings for melons, grapes, and pineapples, which were out of season and hard to obtain. She ate green peppers, tomatoes, croutons, lettuce, and carrots with Thousand Island dressing, but only early in the afternoon. Italian dressing was not an acceptable substitute! On one occasion when she craved Japanese food, her husband took her to a favorite restaurant, an event she eagerly anticipated. Once she was inside the door, waves of nausea forced her to dash outside. She vomited on the street, to the disgust of entering patrons, including an old boyfriend! Another time, her husband took her to a marvelous restaurant atop a Boston skyscraper. Once seated, she was unable to eat because the restaurant was filled with what she described as "heavy fall food smells all around." Her nausea had started during the journey to the top floor in the high-speed elevator. This was a trigger she was not expecting. No one had ever mentioned that riding in an elevator might effect her, and this was the first time she had ridden in such a contraption when pregnant.

Events like these constantly caught her unawares and left her dejected.

She was unable to eat beef or eggs, formerly among her favorite foods. Turkey sandwiches, however, were benign enough that she could eat them without getting sick. As she put it, "Turkey doesn't have much smell or taste anyway." The foods she found consistently "safe" were potato chips, cold fruit, sweet "textured" cake and cookies, chocolate ice cream, strawberries, masala tea, and white toast with butter.

The *masala* tea was something she'd never tried before she became pregnant. One day, a good friend from India visited her with a few tea bags of this highly seasoned and aromatic tea as a gift. Initially Amy recoiled—mostly at the thought of something spicy—but upon tasting the iced tea her friend prepared, she discovered that she liked it. Her friend explained that some women in India drink it for morning sickness. The ingredients include black tea, ginger, cinnamon, black pepper, cloves, and cardamon. Amy thought it strange and interesting that different cultures have different solutions for the same problem.

She commented that as her morning sickness continued past the "magic first trimester mark" when the mother-to-be is *supposed* to feel better, her husband became more and more distant. She later discovered that he felt ill himself whenever she vomited. He felt entirely responsible for her morning sickness and experienced an overwhelming sense of helplessness and hopelessness. When he left the scene during her bouts of vomiting, he felt better physically but emotionally very guilty.

The smells that triggered Amy's nausea and vomiting included food smells, especially the odor of the gravy from Salisbury steak and garlic bread. "Body" smells, especially perfume, were destabilizing factors even though she knew she was smelling "smells no one else could smell." Cigarette smoke, she said, went right to her stomach, but for some strange reason she could tolerate the smoke from the burning logs in her father-in-law's fireplace fairly well. The taste of plain water would precipitate vomiting, but drinking ice-cold, unsweetened iced tea (like the masala tea) left her feeling "just fine." So she continued to drink it to the end of her pregnancy. She could never figure out ahead of time when plain tea would work better than masala, which she called "high test." "I have to trust my gut—ha ha!!—when I get to that decision point of having 10 seconds to decide what to go for to keep this monster [morning sickness] controlled!"

In March, when she delivered a full-term, healthy baby girl, Amy's weight was 165 pounds, only 15 pounds above her prepregnancy weight.

MAGGIE AND TED

A man whose wife endured morning sickness during two pregnancies, Ted found his relatives' comments the most difficult part of the experience to survive. During the second pregnancy, the couple's first child, Scotty, was often cared for by Maggie's mother. But *his* mother, a very traditional woman, was horrified that her daughter-in-law was not cooking dinners for Scotty, who ate cold cereal and milk most nights. The family gossiped, whispering, "Oh, she can't be that sick!" Only when Maggie ended up in the hospital with major complications due to gallbladder disease in pregnancy, on top of severe morning sickness, did other family members recognize the serious nature of her ordeal.

Their second baby, Lance, weighed in at 7 pounds, 3 ounces. But Maggie's predelivery weight was 40 pounds less than her prepregnancy weight of 165 pounds. The stress and strain of the 9-month struggle were evident to everyone who knew "Mags" as a fun-loving, high-energy woman. Eight weeks after Lance was born, Maggie entered the hospital for a 2-day stay to have her gallbladder removed. Ted said it seemed a lot easier for the relatives to understand a gallbladder problem than morning sickness. With the 40-pound weight loss, Maggie's "get up and go" had got up and gone! It took her almost a year to regain back her old vim and vigor.

DEFINING MORNING SICKNESS

The technical name for moderate-to-severe nausea and vomiting during pregnancy is hyperemesis gravidarum (HG). There is another aspect to the definition of HG, it can get so bad that a woman needs to be hospitalized for care. There are many shades of gray between moderate and severe morning sickness. Currently, there is no set of criteria that can delineate this spectrum.

Personally, I have encountered women on postpartum units who have told me horror stories of their pregnancies—losing 10 to 20 pounds, losing lots of work time, and receiving intravenous fluids at their doctors' offices or seeking care in emergency rooms. I would call a woman who fits this description of 24/7 morning sickness a *hyperemetic*. How this woman would be coded in the medical data collection system, I have no idea—and that, I think, is a problem. (How a woman's insurance company sees weight loss in pregnancy is an entirely different issue that no one has looked at yet.)

The classical obstetrical definition of hyperemesis gravidarum is

1. A weight loss of 5 percent or more with ketosis (when ketones are produced by the body's breakdown of fat for energy)

2. Retinal (eye), renal (kidney), or hepatic (liver) damage
3. Neurological alteration
4. Intractable vomiting and disturbed nutrition

This definition was established in 1956 by the American Counsel on Pharmacy and Chemistry and is still the working criteria for determining when a woman should be admitted to the hospital for care. These guidelines do not provide examples of how much retinal, renal, or hepatic damage is the threshold, nor do they really define *neurological alteration*.

As the above stories also illustrate, morning sickness effects the lives not only of pregnant women but often of their spouses and the rest of their families. It can combine some or all of the following symptoms, for different durations and at various levels of intensity:

Nausea, vomiting, and retching

Aversion to odors (some of which previously might have been considered pleasant)

Aversion to bright lights

Aversion to loud noises

Aversion to snug-fitting clothes

Sensitivity to invasion of personal space (perhaps better described as low-level claustrophobia)

Sensitivity to visual motion from computer screens that flicker, television images, or poor-quality video images with grainy texture

See Table 1.1 for more symptoms of morning sickness compiled from common medical literature and my personal experience in practice. When events are severe and uncontrolled early, it appears likely that the course of morning sickness (hyperemesis) can be prolonged and become more severe.

Table 1.1 Symptoms of Morning Sickness

Mild	Severe
Nausea with or without vomiting–worse in the morning upon rising*	Nausea and vomiting, not limited to a specific time
Possible weight loss	Weight loss over 5% between 5–8 weeks *
Intolerance of cold	Intolerance of cold
Possible constipation	Constipation
Ability to eat between periods of nausea	Difficulty eating or drinking
Ability to fall asleep	Difficulty falling asleep (but relief often comes with sleep)
Appropriate urine output	Limited and highly concentrated urine output
Lying down helpful	Lying down more helpful in a dark, quiet room
Tiredness (avoiding fatigue extremely important in reducing nausea)	Extreme fatigue (may often wake from a nap because of nausea)
Symptoms triggered by heat or cold	Nausea aggravated by physical temperature extremes
	Inability to perform activities of daily living
	At least one trip to an emergency room in the first eight weeks *
	Blood electrolyte levels abnormal, indicating dehydration and starvation (changes in potassium, magnesium, and phosphorous in particular)
	Ketone positive readings (This indicates that stored fat is being burned due to energy intake being below biological needs. Aggressive hydration will reduce this, potentially only temporarily.)
	Slow or impaired thinking
	An increase in saliva resulting in difficulty swallowing
	Decreased attention span

Table 1.1   Symptoms of Morning Sickness *(continued)*

Severe

Decreased motivation

Decreased physical performance

Increased anxiety

Boredom

Symptoms aggravated by motions
(This can be either visual motion,
like TV close-ups and rapid scene
changes or physical motion, like
stop-and-go motion of a car.)

Poor skin tone

Dry, shrunken tongue

Aching eyeballs, difficulty focusing
with rapid visual changes

Occasional thoughts about drastic
options, especially termination;
occasional fleeting suicide thoughts*

Need for aggressive medical
nutrition therapy, either tube
feeding or intravenous nutrition
(This is referred to as total parental
nutrition)*

*These are criteria the author has established based on symptoms of the large number of women she has treated.

It's Not Just in the Morning

In spite of the name, morning sickness doesn't attack only in the morning. Like the symptoms of morning sickness, which vary from woman to woman, the time of day at which the ailment hits is different for each expectant mother. In a study conducted on 244 women in the first trimester, 50 percent felt sickest mainly in the morning. Less than 10 perent felt sickest either in the evening or in both the morning and the evening. Roughly 33 percent felt sick all day long, and about one in eight had such severe nausea and vomiting during the whole day that ordinary activity was impossible.

If you are one of those women whose symptoms occur primarily in the morning, it may be because of a sudden transition from sleeping to wakefulness. Abrupt motions, such as reaching to turn off a noisy alarm clock, can disturb your equilibrium. As you start to move around at the beginning of the day, you may feel increased awareness of negative sensations. Even the movement of a restless bed partner can contribute to the morning sickness of pregnancy. Avoiding these "morning triggers" may help you deal with your first bouts of sickness during the day.

How Long Does It Last?

There's a popular assumption that morning sickness goes away at the end of the first trimester, that is, by the thirteenth week of the pregnancy. This idea has been disproved by several well-controlled studies. In one involving 414 pregnant women, the research found that 10.6 percent reported no symptoms. In contrast to this cohort were the 86.5 percent who experienced nausea and the 53 percent who experienced vomiting with nausea. Of the women who suffered from nausea in early pregnancy, about 25 percent were still having it at week 20. An unspecified but significant number continued to feel nauseated until the end of the pregnancy. This study showed the average duration of morning sickness was 17.3 weeks, which is about 4 weeks longer than most doctors and books cite.

When I interview pregnant and postpartum women, many say their nausea subsided at 4 or 5 months. However, I have also spoken with and cared for women whose nausea, with intermittent vomiting, continued to the day of delivery. A study from South Africa indicated that 5 percent of women are sick to term. An Australian report speculated that 20 percent of all women with nausea and vomiting continue to suffer to the end of their pregnancies—not a pleasant prospect. However, being aware of these statistics may be helpful for some women when the weeks come and go and the nausea and vomiting don't.

Women, their families, and their doctors often express frustration about trying to cope with the nausea and vomiting of morning sickness because of the unpredictable waxing and waning of symptoms. There may be a few great days between bouts when everyone begins to think life is back to normal. Often, once a woman starts to feel better after a seemingly endless period of being sick, she tackles waiting projects with a vengeance. But morning sickness can recur without warning.

Some people are not ready for all the changes that severe or prolonged morning sickness will impose on them. For example, because morning sickness is so unpredictable, you may need to think about any travel plans you consider taking before your baby is born (the "last get-aways"). The factors involved with traveling, as you may recall from previous trips, include long lines, smells of perfume or cologne, cigarette smoke, crowds, food smells on airlines, mystery meals, or no food! All of these routine challenges take on a very different dimension when you add them to chronic nausea. Also, severe air turbulance is always possible. If you end up being extremely sick on your flight, you might end up in an unfamiliar hospital on the road. If you decide at the airport that you just can't get on board, you may risk losing your money unless you bought cancellation insurance coverage. A note from your doctor that says you are queasy and green won't cut it with the financial department at the airline headquarters!

IF YOU ARE MISERABLE, YOU ARE NOT ALONE

Every woman with morning sickness has probably heard, "Try tea, toast, or JELL-O." "Don't think about it, and it'll go away." "Did you try eating crackers?" For many women, this sort of advice isn't worth much. If you're suffering from fairly severe morning sickness, you undoubtedly feel exhausted and alone in your constant debilitating nausea. But you shouldn't, because literally millions of women every year share your predicament. Fifty to ninety percent of all women have some degree of gastrointestinal discomfort in early pregnancy. For some women, the morning nausea subsides as the day goes on. However, several studies point out that between 36 and 76 percent of all women feel sick all day long, especially in the first trimester.

This is not anecdotal information: A research nurse investigated the degree of nausea and vomiting of 133 women in five different obstetrical practices in Boston. All the pregnancies were at week 20 or earlier. Less than 10 percent of the women had not been nauseated at all in the 2 days before they visited their doctors. Twenty-three percent had been nauseated from 3 to 6 hours during the 2-day period, 15 percent from 7 to 15 hours, 10 percent from 13 to 18 hours, and 17 percent more than 18 hours. These same women were also asked to rate the severity of their nausea in the 2 days before their visits to the doctor. Slightly over 33 percent described their nausea as "mild," 56 percent called it "moderate," and 7 percent considered the nausea "severe." When asked to report the number of times they had vomited, slightly less than two-thirds said they had had not vomited at all in the past two days, 27 percent had vomited from one to three times, 8 percent had vomited from four to six times, and 3 percent had vomited more than six times.

Thankfully the study did not find any correlation of adverse outcome with the varying episodes of vomiting. The healthiness of the pregnancy did not seem to be linked to the degree of sickness the women felt. Because no one was hospitalized in this study, no one was classified as having hyperemesis gravidarum.

Every woman responds to morning sickness in her own way. You may be more afflicted with vomiting than with nausea. If you've had previous problems with motion sickness, gastric distress, migraine headaches, and adverse reactions to birth control pills, your nausea may be more intense. For many women, morning sickness may be their first experience with feeling under the weather for any extended period of time.

RELAPSE

If a woman experiences a new cycle of nausea, vomiting, or both, it probably stems from a combination of factors. These include continuing hormonal fluctuations and probably a number of external triggers, which will be discussed later. Often the relapse is set off by a major "trigger," usually a smell. To avoid a relapse, you need to avoid culprit smells, noise, and bright light. You may also have to refrain from major activities, such as commuting to work, cleaning house, and attending parties (especially those that feature copious amounts of aromatic foods). One way to get through this time is to use trial and error to find foods that can break the nausea and vomiting cycle. (See Chapter 9, "Managing Morning Sickness with Food" for more details.) It's difficult not to get discouraged and angry during this time, but "the miserables" do go away eventually, even if it the end is not until the baby is born!

MY ULTIMATE WISH LIST

Walking to work years ago, I saw a vacant, bright yellow, Southern colonial-type mansion on Kent Street in Brookline. This place spoke to me. It said, "I should become the Miriam Halfway House for Hyperemetics"! (Wouldn't that be great?)

The MHWHH would provide a bump-reduced limo ride to and from local airports. The drivers would be trained medics dressed as limo chauffeurs. The kitchen would be in the attic—reducing food smells. We would install direct phone lines to local stores and eateries to provide for instant grocery and take-out food delivery. There would be patio dining outside on first floor and lots of watermelon and lemonade available in the spring and summer. There would be a fenced-in front yard for kids coming to visit, and child-development majors from local colleges would be on hand to provide expert day care. There would be foot massages for evening relaxation. The facility would be close to several local hospitals if the need for hospitalization arose.

In Dreamland, admissions to the halfway house would be covered by insurance because it would be cheaper than a hospital admission. It would be a three-part combination: 1/3 hospital, 1/3 outpatient/day care, and 1/3 inn. I, of course, would be the director!

Unfortunately, it doesn't look like I'll luck into that piece of real estate or that dream job anytime soon, so this book will need to be a proxy.

Chapter 2

How Morning Sickness Affects Women and Their Families

BETSY

After being admitted three times for overnight stays in the emergency room for hydration, Betsy finally landed for a prolonged stay on a hospital gynecology unit. She was 5 1/2 weeks pregnant with twins. This was her second pregnancy; she was 37 years old. She told one of her health care providers that she had lost her first baby at the beginning of her second trimester 14 years earlier, at age 23, because of constant nausea, vomiting, and poor nutrition. The nurse noted this information and thought it was curious because she recalled that the medical literature asserts that morning sickness does not usually result in spontaneous termination, especially in very early pregnancy and to young women.

Once she was comfortable with her care providers, Betsy mentioned that she was no stranger to the hospital. During her first pregnancy 14 years ago, she had been admitted to the emergency room of a large hospital in another state "about a dozen times" and had also endured one or two stays on a patient care unit. During that first pregnancy, although she was treated immediately because of her emergency case status, she considered the care she received ineffective. Her main complaint was that her relief was always short-lived. In addition, she felt as if she was always "bothering someone." She described her prior experience with medical caregivers: "I thought they all looked at me like I was some sort of freak because I just never got over the nausea and vomiting like they said I would at 12 weeks."

During one of her hospitalizations in her first pregnancy, when the overworked antenatal staff was totally frustrated and felt they had nothing more to offer Betsy, they called in a psychiatrist. After he examined her, Betsy was stunned to overhear him mumbling that she was "probably vomiting just to upset the nurses." At one point she was given Tigan, an antinausea medication, in suppository form. When she complained of lower abdominal cramping and started vomiting again, an exhausted resident was called to evaluate the situation at 2:00 a.m. He examined her and left, and then returned about 10 minutes later with a small tube. He stated that the only solution to her lack of nutrition was tube feeding. He explained the tube he held needed to be inserted through her nose, then it would go down the esophagus and into her stomach. Once the tube was in place, she would be hooked up to a machine that would dispense a formula to provide complete fluid and nutrition. That sounded great, but the sensation of the thin tube being inserted into her nasal passage produced an uncomfortable sensation. Not wanting to appear uncooperative, Betsy allowed him to attempt to insert the tube into her nose, without benefit of nasal Xylocaine, an anesthetic agent. Betsy began to retch and cry. Betsy tried to explain that she was about vomit, but the warning was too late. She vomited yellow-green bile on the resident's lab coat. This ended the tube-feeding effort. In the morning, the resident said, another doctor would be around to decide what alternative courses should be considered.

The thoughts running through Betsy's head were desperate, "Is it worth having a baby?" "How can I love a baby who is making me this miserable?" "What will happen if I hate this kid?" "I can't possibly deal with someone sticking something in my nose again. I'll lose my mind over this!" Betsy finally fell asleep at 3:00 a.m., vowing that she would be out of hospital in the morning. She was certain that being sick at home was preferable to what was in store for her at the hospital. She was wrong. The morning sickness just got worse. She could not cope anymore.

During her second pregnancy, her doctor contacted Betsy's former care provider and learned through transfer records that she had decided to terminate her first pregnancy after 11 weeks of constant nausea and vomiting, no sleep or relief, the traumatic emergency room episode, and ultimately the loss of her job. A psychiatric note in her records from the first pregnancy suggested she might have had a conversion disorder (you'll learn more about this later in the chapter.) She was reported to have been acting quite bizarre on several occasions. An entry from a registered dietitian commented on her 8 percent weight loss and the need to consider intervention for nutrition. That was the last clinical notation before Betsy's discharge and the subsequent termination of her pregnancy.

Fourteen years later, Betsy was overwhelmed by the surprise news of her twin pregnancy. During her subsequent hospital admission, she said, "I hope it doesn't happen again." Her nurse thought she meant the morning sickness, but in fact Betsy was thinking about the termination of her previous pregnancy and worrying about having enough stamina to endure what might be weeks of misery. Twins, a new husband, a new stepdaughter—there was a lot on Betsy's mind.

Betsy had recently moved to New England with her second husband, Joe, because of his new job, and she hoped she was ready to make a fresh start and try to start a family again. In the big metropolitan hospital she was admitted to during the second pregnancy, she learned that other women were also hospitalized with debilitating morning sickness routinely on the high-risk pregnancy unit. She was relieved. Just knowing that she was not crazy and not alone made a huge difference in her feelings about being sick all the time.

But the second pregnancy was also punctuated by several emergency room admissions for hydration therapy. Joe and his teenage daughter from a previous marriage, Tess, accompanied her on some visits. On one occasion Tess had commented she thought that when she grew up she would like to have several children. However, watching Betsy gag, retch, vomit, eventually collapse, and end up in the hospital forced her to rethink that decision: "I'm not sure anymore! Granted, Betsy hasn't been my favorite person up to now. We both know that, but I can't stand to see her go through this. The gagging noises make me want to chuck! Most of my family thinks she's making it up, but I see her retching over the toilet at night—when I'm having a weekend over. She's trying to be quiet, but I hear her puking and crying at 2:00 in the morning. Then she cleans herself up and tries to look cheerful in the morning like nothing happened. I know she doesn't want to upset my Dad. I never asked him how he feels about this pregnancy—was it his idea or not? Would he care if she just quit it? I want to ask her so many questions, but I just don't know how."

Tess continued to talk about how Betsy's illness affected her family, "When Dad told me that I'd have a brother or sister I was really irked because Dad would have another kid in his new life . . . and I thought I wouldn't matter. Then I got excited when Bet said I could pick out the stroller and help with decorating the baby's bedroom. A few of my friends' mothers have had babies recently, but I can't remember one story of a puke-a-thon going on for months! I worry she's going to die. . . . I worry that they'll get divorced over it. . . . They both look so unhappy! Are these Franken-kids?—Some sort of monsters?"

Betsy never discussed her morning sickness with Tess because she was worried it might impact the girl's future family plans. As for Joe, the prospect of having three kids was stress enough. She knew he was working overtime already to pay for extra help to cook for her and clean the house. So she avoided discussing her discomfort with him as well.

She was worried about Tess and Joe, but she needed to focus on her own problems. She'd discovered an Internet abortion support group and began to chat online with people who could help her understand that her former choice really had nothing to do with her current situation. She learned to believe that she was not being punished for a decision she had made years before when she was woefully uninformed about her choices. E-mail by e-mail, Betsy promised her online friends that she would get through another day, no matter what. Despite the encouragement she received, her weight was dropping, and her spirits were up and down.

She was learning to live with the chronic nausea and getting some relief with much psychological encouragement and intravenous home fluid support. Thankful for all the help she was getting this time around, she decided that she wanted to "give back." So Betsy made herself available in Internet chat rooms to other women suffering from morning sickness. Providing suggestions and chatting with other women in similar dire straits was a relief for her as well as to the women she "spoke" with. The most important thing that she learned during her visits to online chat rooms was that hundreds of women are in this situation every year, and many were going through it all alone. Providing (and receiving) love and support to women she never even met personally really made a difference to her.

Of course, figuring out what foods she could tolerate was an important part of Betsy's pregnant life. One favorite food item during her second pregnancy was the diet soda Fresca, something she'd never tried before her illness. Her responses to different foods and beverages kept changing. She found the odd combination of raspberry ginger ale and Reese's peanut butter cups successful for a few days. Then she found that she couldn't eat anything except pasta for a day or two.

During the 9 long months of her pregnancy, Betsy's doctor saw her often as an add-on emergency case for hydration therapy in his office. At 28 weeks, she was still sick. Betsy and her doctor worked out this arrangement because he was tired of being called in the middle of the night by the emergency room staff at the hospital. Betsy tried her best to keep her sense of humor through all this misery. She'd check in with the receptionists saying, "Well, here I am again, Prego, Puko Patty!" Betsy kept a diary of events and found that many of her really bad days occurred one day ahead of incoming bad weather and the accompanying barometric pressure lows and disturbances.

Finally, the babies were born, full-term and healthy at 39 weeks. Betsy decided to breastfeed to take advantage of all the motherhood experiences she could. As she put it, "These kiddos are worth it, but no more! As much as we all love them, none of us can imagine doing this again."

MORNING SICKNESS AND YOUR MENTAL AND PHYSICAL WELL-BEING

Morning sickness can affect women in many different ways. It also can affect their families profoundly. In this chapter, we will discuss some of the ways mornings sickness can manifest itself—from the physical to the emotional. In the following chapters, we will discuss in more detail the effects of morning sickness on the mind and the body and various ways you can attempt to alleviate some of its worst symptoms.

CONVERSION DISORDER

After reading about Betsy, you may be wondering just what a *conversion disorder* is. It's a psychiatric term for the acute onset of sensory or motor symptoms that are unexplained by physical findings. Basically, it is used to describe someone who is physically ill or depressed and disoriented for no easily detectable, common medical reason. Years ago, it was believed to be associated with a hysterical personality, but thankfully that notion has been dispelled in modern times.

There is a paper in the medical literature describing three cases of women with conversion disorder and morning sickness. What all three of these case studies have in common is that the women suffered from weeks of nausea, vomiting, and weight loss. Woman A lost 20 pounds, and Woman B lost 16 pounds. No weight-loss data was provided for Woman C. From this information we can assume that these women were pretty malnourished. Motor impairment, moodiness, anxiety, and depression also often accompany malnutrition and sleep deprivation. If your physician mentions conversion disorder to you, it means that you are suffering from a number of serious symptoms that will affect you both physically and mentally.

VISION PROBLEMS

Some women who wear contact lenses find that the lenses get uncomfortable during pregnancy. This may be caused by rising estrogen levels, which can cause fluid retention and affect the shape of the cornea. Unfortunately, it appears that with estrogen fluxes and changes in hydration status, the shape of the eye can change ever so slightly, resulting in eye discomfort and visual changes that can act as a trigger for morning sickness.

This might be the reason that looking at computer screens and some florescent lights makes some pregnant women a bit queasy. Even some fabric patterns, such as hounds-tooth check and paisley, can create a visual feeling of motion. If the eye is sending motion signals to the brain and the stomach, this may be why some women feel better in quiet dark rooms.

THE SALIVA THING

Many women complain of bitter-tasting saliva or copious amounts of it when suffering from morning sickness. Some even say that they feel like a drooling dog! This is more common than you may think. Having done a survey on morning sickness with *Shape/Fit Pregnancy* in 1994, I know from my data that 37 percent of the respondents (113 women) shared this complaint. It seems to be a hallmark of morning sickness for many.

One study suggests that 13 percent of pregnant women experience salivary changes when pregnant. Many described their saliva as thick and milky with a sharp metallic taste or, alternatively, as thin, bubbly, bitter, and watery. Respondents reported that the intensity of saliva volume interfered with interpersonal relationships (43 percent), swallowing (40 percent), taste (33 percent), sleep (30 percent), and speech (30 percent).

The average (nonpregnant) person produces about 1200 cc/day (over a quart) of saliva. Besides containing many electrolytes (sodium, potassium, bicarbonate, magnesium), saliva also is full of growth factors. Growth factors are protein substances produced by the body that are important for the normal growth and development of various cells. At this time, researchers are beginning to learn that certain disease states—Alzheimer's and Parkinson's diseases, for example—have reduced levels of growth-associated proteins. The growth factors found in saliva are likely to be important for normal cell health in the stomach.

Progesterone is responsible for the viscosity (thickness) of saliva, whereas gastric acid appears to affect its volume (quantity). When gastric acids (the acid your stomach produces to digest food) come in contact with the esophagus, salivation increases. This is probably a protective function, because saliva is basic and gastric contents are acidic. So the basic nature of the saliva protects our organs from stomach acids that might harm them.

Some foods seem to increase saliva production; dairy products, followed by protein foods, top the list. Fruits, grains, and vegetables have been shown not to have a huge adverse effect on saliva production. The majority of women with this problem report that lemon or ginger drinks reduce the bitter taste in their mouths, whereas cool solids (such as ice cream or frozen fruit bars) seem to lessen the excessive fluid production.

MORNING SICKNESS AND YOUR CAREER

Professional and high-powered career women seem to have more difficulty coping with the newly acquired disability of nausea and vomiting because they regard themselves as "super women." Used to 60-plus hour work weeks and three nights per week at the gym, the loss of control and the feeling of not being as physically fit as usual may be devastating to these women. Many women who work on a bonus system as part of their income feel especially devastated by morning sickness. Often they have not told co-workers of being pregnant for fear of office politics. More than one woman I have cared for has lost her job because she has taken too many sick days.

I took care of a woman in the recent past who was fired because she missed work too many times because of her hyperemesis. Previous to that, she had an outstanding work record. Even though her physicians provided documentation of her disability, her immediate boss was unhelpful. He hadn't encountered hyperemesis gravidarum previously and was not about to become educated on the subject. This woman had planned to return to work as soon as possible after she had her baby. She was furious about being terminated and hired a lawyer to sue for wrongful dismissal. Her case is currently undecided.

PREGNANCY DISABILITY ACT

The Pregnancy Disability Act is an amendment to Title VII of the Civil Rights Act of 1964. Discrimination on the basis of pregnancy, childbirth, or related medical conditions constitutes unlawful sex discrimination under Title VII. Employers must treat pregnant women the same as any other person otherwise temporarily disabled. That said, this disability act does not address morning sickness directly. For more information about the Pregnancy Disability Act, check out www.eeoc.gov/facts/fs-preg.html.

MORNING SICKNESS AND YOUR FAMILY

Not much research has been published to date on the effect morning sickness has on families, but it is a major concern of sick women. Women report to me that toddlers often pat moms on the back as they are hanging over toilet bowls and then go on to empathetically "gag" along side. Older children will remember more of the events of seeing a woman in bed for weeks, not being happy with being pregnant. Some women will talk about it and tell their children that it's temporary. Some women do not talk about it because they do not know what to say.

This section offers some considerations for parents and health care providers who are dealing with the effects of morning sickness on the family. (These have been adapted from my communication with Dr. Shari Munch, assistant professor of social work at Rutgers University in New Jersey and perinatal social worker.) A mother's illness usually creates a crisis for the family. The mother is often the "glue" of the family. When she is not around, for whatever reason, lots of things fall apart. You'll find a change in roles. The husband or partner must take on the mother's responsibilities—like it or not—whether he's been taught what they are or not! Actually, it is a smart idea for a woman who is sick to jot down the (enormous) list of "mom responsibilities" just to reduce the trial-by-fire initiation. Older children often are given more responsibility and asked to help out with household chores. Some children may resent this because they are staying home more and worry about becoming socially isolated from peers. Many women who work outside the home may have housekeepers, nannies, and whatever other services keep a household in motion and functioning. When there's a lack of money coming into the household because of missed work due to morning sickness, some of these services may come to a screeching halt. However, whether they work outside the home or not, women are typically in charge of grocery shopping and feeding the family. A sick mom might end up on the couch or at the hospital. As a result, food procurement plans can also change, which can wreak havoc in any family.

Young children may be especially confused and saddened to be separated from their primary caretaker (if mom is the primary caretaker). They often are shuffled from a variety of care providers (e.g., relatives, neighbors, day care centers), disrupting their normal routines. Even children who are used to being in day care situations expect to see their mothers at some point in the day. When mom is not there to pick them up at the end of the day, it may result in worry and stress for both mom and the kids.

Young children may demonstrate regressive behaviors. For example, if they are already potty-trained, they may begin to wet the bed again. This can result in extra stress and work (washing bedclothes every day) and may be very frustrating for parents and caregivers. Even if this is the case, punishment is not advised! This is a coping behavior—a reaction to stress. Young children at this age are not able to articulate their feelings; thus, stress may manifest itself in behavioral changes. It's important for parents and any other caregivers to remember that temporary behavioral transgressions such as bed-wetting should not be punished at this time. Be sure to talk about any behavioral reactions to stress your child may be having with anyone you leave your child with, and be sure to send along an extra set of sheets, absorbent pads, diapers, or training pants as well!

Young children may need to hear that their "magical thinking" didn't cause mom's illness. Children may have internal worries that their thoughts about not wanting the baby have caused their mother's illness.

Children may worry about whether their mother might die from this. This is the case especially if their mother is in hospital or at home with invasive intervention (e.g., nasogastric [NG] tube, intravenous nutrition, or Reglan pump with intravenous lines).

Older children may be jealous about the fact that a new person will soon be coming to live in their house, especially if they have been the king or queen of the roost for some time. If their house is cramped to begin with, they might be angry that they will have to share space with an "invader." They may say insensitive things because of it. They may even be embarrassed that their mom is pregnant! The unavoidable realization that their mother has had sex might really be a shock to their systems. Older children, especially female teenagers, worry that this will happen to them when they decide to get pregnant. All of these feelings may result in additional resentment towards the illness that is affecting the sanctuary of their home.

For expectant mothers with children, I strongly suggest family or spiritual counseling to try to minimize confusion and stress. In addition, here are some other things you can do to help your children. Make sure to stay involved with your kids even if you are ill or hospitalized. Phone calls can be as important as physical visits if you are in the hospital. Young children can draw pictures to hang in your bedroom or hospital room. Make an effort to hang photos of children in your bedroom or hospital room so that when they spend time with you they can see how important and special they are to you. Let kids get into bed with you (if you can tolerate it) and read books or watch television with them. If, like many sick moms, you find "jiggling bed syndrome" to be aggravating, work with your children to get through it together. Call it JBS and tell your child that the treatment for this is for them to sneak quietly into your bed and be very gentle when they cuddle you. You can say, "I have JBS: jiggling bed syndrome. Any jiggling of the bed might make me sick. That's why I have to be very still and quiet. Can you help me by being as quiet as a baby mouse and as still as a baby deer in the forest?"

It's important to tell your kids the medical facts. Make sure you provide them with age-appropriate information. For example you might say, "Mommy is sick, and her sickness is called HG. That's why mommy throws up a lot. She'll be better as soon as the baby comes." Even if young kids do not fully understand, they need to hear the term HG (for hyperemesis gravidarum) so that if they have a stomachache or throw up or don't feel like eating, they won't think that they have HG. This way, you help them learn to differentiate between various types of sickness. Also, show even very young kids the tubes. Tell them what the tubes do and that they are there to help. Children might be afraid to approach you with an NG tube in your nose. Providing positive information about how the doctors are helping you (rather than hurting) is important.

If your child plays with dolls, it's possible that your child will try to create tubes for the doll that are similar to yours. Don't be surprised if you see a drinking straw taped to the doll's nose or arm.

Keep your children's routine as normal as possible (bedtime, meals, activities, school, etc.). Try to place them with caregivers they trust and know, if possible. Avoid overrelying on teenagers to take on excessive responsibilities; they need to have their own lives, too.

Allow expression of feelings—sadness, crying, and so forth. Don't forget the obvious: Give lots of love and hugs if you can. Hugs can be difficult if you have "radar nose." The smell of a child's breath or a wet diaper can be a set back. Hugs can also sometimes be tricky if you have many lines and tubes attached to your body. You may be worried that they will be pulled out or twisted. If you can't provide a real hug, give a hug gift certificate to be redeemed at the first opportunity. Or, in lieu of a hug, other touching, such as hair braiding or face painting, might be an effective alternative.

REJECTION

Dr. Munch has counseled moms who were upset that their young kids (1 to 3 years old) ignored them or seemed aloof when they visited their mother at the hospital. Sometimes this continues even when mothers return home from the hospital. Rest assured that this is normal. Very young children will attach to whatever person is most consistently there for them. If mom is gone, they will become closest to dad or other more present caregivers. Unfortunately, this can be especially painful for mothers. You just need to know that it might happen and that it is developmentally normal. Once you are feeling better and are back at home more, the kids will come around again.

CULTURAL AND GENERATIONAL ISSUES

With any family, there are cultural differences that may come into the picture. How other people handle children, crises, and stress might well be different from how your family handles things. If you have difficulty talking about these issues with your child-care providers, be sure to contact a licensed social worker to help you and your family figure out a positive strategy to get through this difficult time.

Every mother and her family will probably react differently to disability, hospitalization, and illness. They will deal with the situation in terms of their own unique family dynamics, personalities, spiritual beliefs, and ethnic or racial background. We can't say that all Asian-American families will react alike any more than all the families in your neighborhood will, whether you live in New York City, Saigon, or rural Maine. Expect to encounter generational issues, too, if grandparents are called upon to provide emergency child care. Their child-rearing beliefs, especially those surrounding a reward and punishment system may not be similar to yours.

COUVADE SYNDROME

Couvade syndrome, affecting the spouses of some pregnant women, has been around for a long time. Plutarch describes it in documents dating from 60 B.C. The word *couvade* comes from the Basque verb meaning to brood or hatch. In a study conducted in upstate New

York of 300 couples, there were 267 men who agreed to be studied. Of this group, 60 men (22.5%) had Couvade syndrome as defined by the researchers. These men had physical symptoms unexplained by events other than their wives being pregnant.

According to one researcher, men who experienced Couvade had more visits before their wives' pregnancy to see a medical professional as well as after the pregnancy than men without Couvade. Interestingly, the men in the study who were found to have Couvade syndrome had had twice the number of medical visits during the pregnancy as before. The symptoms they complained of were nausea, vomiting, abdominal pain, and abdominal bloating. These men were concerned with their appetite, weight, bowel changes, leg cramps, faintness, and lassitude.

Findings from a 3-year study conducted by Dr. Jacqueline Clinton of the University of Wisconsin Milwaukee School of Nursing showed that men with Couvade syndrome also complained of morning sickness, fatigue, backaches, depression, insomnia, increased stress, weight gain, and cravings for particular foods. Dr. Clinton studied 147 husbands of expectant women from ages 18 to 45 who had no disabilities, chronic pain, or mental illness. These men were matched with a control goup of 66 men who were not expectant fathers. The most common complaint reported in the study was short-temperedness—not only with the person's wife but with strangers.

Chapter 3

Why Do We Get Morning Sickness?

CARRIE

A successful woman with her own business, Carrie had received hospital treatment twice previously for the same problem: morning sickness. Before the official confirmation of her second pregnancy, Carrie knew she was pregnant. One day while dressing her son, she became acutely aware that the baby "smelled." The smell, she said, was not unclean, just "a real strong people smell." She also noticed that her laundry now smelled to her of heavy perfume, but she had changed neither her detergent nor her method of laundering. Clothes from the cleaners also had a new distinct chemical odor.

Carrie's nausea progressed to vomiting about 7 1/2 weeks into her pregnancy, and her weight dropped 10 pounds. Her doctor decided hospitalization was necessary the day she collapsed in her office. What she did not tell her doctor was that the previous week she had taken a 2-hour flight to an important business meeting. The plane experienced about 20 minutes of very turbulent air, rendering Carrie hopelessly sick in a first-class lavatory for an extended period of time—irritating fellow travelers. In an attempt to avoid just this scenario, she had purposely bought an expensive first-class seat to avoid food smells from other travelers, but she hadn't counted on a bad flight. She was so weak at the end of the flight that the flight attendant insisted she leave the plane in a wheelchair. Needless to say, she had to cancel her meeting.

During her hospital stay, Carrie had a slightly green-yellow complexion (jaundice), which seemed to get worse as the days went on, and she was unable to eat or drink. Her doctor was a bit concerned because some of her LFTs (liver function tests) were slightly abnormal. She overheard the doctors on rounds one morning say "the ALT and AST are about two times normal. We'll have to keep an eye on these." In medical lingo, ALT is alanine aminotransferase and AST is asparate aminotransferase, enzymes that are released when there is some organ damage. Starvation can cause increases in liver enzymes, as can some medications, intravenous nutrition if administered too aggressively, and medical problems such as alcoholism and diabetes. Gallbladder problems can also raise LFT's and, in Carrie's case, gallstones were one of the conditions her doctors wanted to rule out. An ultrasound of her right upper quadrant (RUQ)—the space under her right rib cage—revealed sludge, which is basically thick bile. The liver produces bile, which helps break down dietary fat. Bile is normal; sludge is not.

When sludge thickens drastically, it eventually contributes to gallstones. Gallstones are like snowballs going down hill; they start off small and grow in size. When a gallstone gets struck in the common bile duct, the tube that drains bile out of the gallbladder into the upper intestinal tract, bile produced in the liver backs up and causes damage to surrounding organs, including the liver and the pancreas. Other conditions can contribute to an increased risk of gallstones: lack of fiber in the diet, inadequate fluids, being female, inflammatory bowel disease, diabetes, rapid weight loss, fasting or starvation, a high-fat diet, and reportedly high levels of estrogen and progesterone, which are common in pregnancy. High levels of estrogen and progesterone decrease the contraction strength of the gallbladder to empty bile normally. Dehydration reduces internal body water, hence bile starts to thicken.

To keep her mind off her misery, Carrie conducted business over the phone. This diversionary activity caused an older British trained nurse to conclude, "she is in here because she only wants a vacation from taking care of her kid! How can she be sick if she can work? Does she look sick to you? When I was in training, we used to put women in dark rooms all alone with their emesis basins! Jolly oh! Didn't that fix them dearies up fast!"

Carrie was discharged after a 7-day hospital stay, with LFTs declining slightly as she began to nibble on salted pretzel sticks and strawberry cream popsicles—foods she referred to as the "brown and pink friends." She still made numerous trips to the emergency room for intravenous fluids because her insurance coverage did not cover home intravenous fluids for pregnancy but would pay if she received them in the hospital. Years previously, she bought health insurance for entrepreneurs based on price but hadn't reviewed the policy in depth since then. What looked like a bargain then was no bargain now, and she regretted not having thought much about the real meaning of benefits before she got pregnant.

She'd once had an adverse reaction to an antinausea medication—a "thick tongue" as she describes—so her doctor was reluctant to use another. Smell management became paramount because it was an instant trigger. Carrie noted that in the late afternoon, around 4:30, she needed to rest in a dark bedroom or she would become violently sick. The slightest fatigue started the downhill spiral. She was occasionally able to return to her office to work for an hour or two. She commented that if she worked for someone else, "they'd probably have fired me long ago."

Visiting Carrie after her baby was born, all the family members displayed absolute enthusiasm and merriment. However, one elderly aunt commented that she wished information about morning sickness had been around when she was pregnant, some 50 years before. As she put it, "I suffered so much! It was like a living hell! That was it for me! Now you know why you only have one cousin! I can still remember one of the meanest nurses on the planet demanding me to get my act together. . . . Oh and I had to clean myself up too!" According to Aunt Lorna, not only did she experience psychologically traumatic emotional care, but the management of severe morning sickness in her case was what she described as "something from Transylvania and beyond!" As bizarre as it sounds, in the early 1940s a woman who suffered from bad nausea and vomiting may be given injections of her husband's blood, with the theory being that there was something inherent in the spouse's blood that could reduce the problem. I know you probably think you just read something unreal, but it is certainly true! Because hyperemesis was considered a "disease of theories" for years, the prevailing theory generated clinical practices. This was not medical management from voodoo men but rather a practice from the United States, if you can believe that!

Aunt Lorna also mentioned that her older cousin, pregnant and very sick in the later 1920s or early 1930s was threatened by her doctor with the application of leeches to various parts of her body if she didn't stop throwing up!

As far as the attitude of Carrie's nurse, sadly, in the middle 1940s that was the standard of care, certainly in the United Kingdom. Elizabeth Tylden was a psychiatric provider who decided to study what she called the "punitive attitude of the staff toward these acutely ill patients" in 1945. "Ward sisters would adjure the patient to 'pull herself together,' doctors would say 'It is entirely up to you to get better,' and the most angry and foul-mouthed ward maid sent to clean up the mess." Dr. Tylden also interviewed a 28-year-old married sick woman, with one previous premature child, who had had a slightly different version of this care: "no vomit bowl, an abusive cleaner-up, and an attractive male registrar saying, 'Pull yourself together.'" This woman decided to terminate her pregnancy and never have more children.

THEORIES, IDEAS, AND HUNCHES

As I've said, morning sickness is not always limited to early pregnancy, and it can be life-threatening. Although there are many theories about the causes of this problem, and no treatment that guarantees relief, any woman afflicted with morning sickness can do a great deal to manage her care.

You and your family, friends, and co-workers should understand that a pregnant woman suffering from nausea and vomiting *is not*

1. An isolated phenomenon
2. Basically neurotic or unhealthy

3. At any increased risk of having a damaged fetus, as long as the condition does not get extreme and escalate into another complication of dehydration and malnutrition

The symptoms of morning sickness are listed in Table 1.1 (from Chapter 1). Many women experience only the "mild" symptoms, but morning sickness can progress from mild to severe. If the sickness becomes so severe that hospitalization is necessary, it is called hyperemesis gravidarum (pronounced "hy-per-em-eh-sis gravid (rhymes with rabid) ar-um").

Why some women get sicker in early pregnancy than others remains a mystery. Over the years many theories have been proposed, modified, and discarded. About a dozen current hypotheses are briefly presented in the following sections, which provide a snapshot of the physiological changes that occur in a woman's body during the pregnancy and may contribute to morning sickness.

LOWERED BLOOD SODIUM

Some researchers suggest that the discomforts of morning sickness may be associated with the biochemical changes that take place in the body of a newly pregnant woman, mainly the lowering of blood sodium. Increases in the levels of hormones start in early pregnancy and cause a number of changes, including an increase in the amount of water in the body, which results in a higher volume of plasma. Plasma is the fluid portion of the blood; red blood cells form the solid red portion. This increase in the fluid proportion of the blood may lower the proportion of sodium, a major mineral. It is speculated that osmoreceptors (nerve endings that can detect alterations in blood compositions) adjust to this biochemical change over time, yet no one has figured out exactly when this might occur. However, low blood sodium can cause nausea, vomiting, and fatigue.

Baroreceptors, also known as stretch receptors, may also play a part in keeping sodium temporarily low. These receptors are found in the walls of the heart and blood vessels. Baroreceptors allow the blood vessels to relax or contract, depending on the influence of certain peptides and hormones. For example, if urine output is low, the baroreceptors might relax so more blood and fluid are directed to the kidneys. A stress response due to adrenaline might cause a constriction of these same blood vessels and reduce blood flow. When blood pressure falls, whether because of vomiting or inadequate consumption of fluid, baroreceptors trigger a set of physiological responses to counteract the drop. A hormone called ADH (antidiuretic hormone, also known as vasopressin) is secreted. It helps the body retain water, and less urine is excreted. However, unless salty foods or beverages are consumed, sodium levels in the body can stay low.

ADJUSTMENT OF THE BRAIN'S CHEMICAL SENSORS

Another explanation focuses on the role that chemoreceptors in the brain may play. Chemoreceptors are nerve endings that can detect changes in the components of the blood, such as sodium, glucose, hormones, and oxygen. It has been speculated that the dramatic rise in many hormones, especially estrogens, that comes with pregnancy precipitates nausea and vomiting in women who adjust more slowly to the increased levels.

METABOLISM OF PREGNANCY HORMONES

There is also a theory that the pregnancy hormones and their by-products put extra stress on the liver, the organ responsible for filtering the blood. Although the liver has a tremendous capacity for work, some researchers believe that it's the additional metabolic stress of pregnancy that causes changes in liver functions and that, in turn, results in nausea and possible vomiting. This hypothesis is supported by research that shows that some women taking oral contraceptives have undergone small changes in their blood chemistries that originate from the liver. Birth-control pills contain various levels of estrogens and progesterone, and some women taking the pills experience nausea and vomiting. Many women eventually adapt to the side effects; those who don't often stop using oral contraceptives.

Research suggests that vitamin C might protect the liver and prevent liver injury. Vitamin C is an antioxidant, which means that it protects against the damaging effects of free radicals. There is a group of researchers from Israel that demonstrated that hyperemesis—severe morning sickness—does generate free radicals. They add additional vitamin C to the intravenous hydration solutions that they give to morning-sickness patients. Whether women with low levels of vitamin C in their diets before pregnancy have worse morning sickness, we don't know.

A few researchers have looked at various hormones to see which ones were elevated during pregnancy. In 1987, a German group found some interesting differences. Looking at 43 healthy women and 74 women sick with hyperemesis, they found that nonsick women produced 95,047 international units (IUs) of human chorionic gonadotropin in 24 hours, whereas the sick group had 86 percent more, or 176,980 IU.

SLOWER EMPTYING OF THE STOMACH

Some prenatal experts report that pregnancy hormones slow down the emptying of the intestinal tract and stomach. It's thought that a more slowly working intestinal tract can cause nausea and may help explain morning sickness. Nausea in pregnancy has actually been shown, by a test called an electrogastrogram, to precede changes in muscular activity in the stomach. Koch, then at Hershey Medical Center, looked at stomach contractions in a group of 32 pregnant women. Twenty-six of these women had nausea (not vomiting) and were pregnant; six were pregnant without nausea, six were postpartum, and four were healthy but not pregnant women. A total of 42 women were examined.

The women in the study had the following characteristics: their average age was 27 years old; onset of nausea was noticed during the fifth week in most subjects; 76 percent had nausea on a daily basis; and 33 percent vomited at least once a day. Three women were sick only in the morning; most of the women experienced nausea throughout the day. Standard electrodes were positioned on the abdomen to record the electrogastrogram (EGG). Three electrotrodes were positioned on the left upper quadrant, which is in the region between the left breast and waistline. These EGGs were performed for 30 to 45 minutes. What these folks showed was interesting: Stomach contractions of 3 cycle per minute (cpm) are normal, hence no one has complaints of nausea.

The pregnant women without nausea had 3 cpm, same as the healthy controls. Of the women with nausea, four had flat-line patterns, meaning no action. Five had very slow rhythms of 1 to 2 cpm, whereas 16 women had fast rhythms of 4 to 8 cpm, and both groups had nausea.

To date, no study has been done in the pharmaceutical world between various medications, dosages, and gastric rhythms. It's hard to believe that these antinausea drugs, antiemetics, can work on all wave forms—flat-wave, slow-wave, and fast-wave rhythms—and produce relief! It is difficult to believe that one size fits all.

We also don't know whether a sick woman's stomach action flip-flops back and forth between slow-wave and fast-wave action. We also don't know how depleted electrolytes and blood chemistries—phosphorous, magnesium, potassium and sodium—affect these stomach electrical situations. We don't know whether heat or cold changes the action or what other therapies impact these waves. We don't know about the effects of stress hormones or of starvation and dehydration.

When I see a woman holding her stomach, my question is "Does your stomach feel better with heat and pressure or motion of rubbing?" Answers are always different. I'd like to know if stomach massage speeds up or slows down the various gastric dysrhythmias. We need a good study!

Rising Hormone Levels

A woman produces more than 30 hormones during her pregnancy. The major hormones increase dramatically in the early weeks. From weeks 4 to 6, the increases in three major hormones amount to a doubling of the total level of hormones in the blood. From weeks 6 to 8, the increases in these three hormones add up to about 50 percent in the total levels of hormones in the blood. From weeks 8 to 10, the hormone levels double again. Weeks 10 to 12 bring a new major increase to a level which stays fairly constant until week 14. At 14 weeks many hormones are present and continue to increase in various amounts. Reportedly, hormone levels begin to taper off at week 16.

Currently, there is not much research looking at *all* pregnancy hormones in various populations of pregnant women because most pregnancies produce healthy children and hormone research is complicated and expensive. For example, dietary habits influence hormone production. A woman's diet before pregnancy may not be consistent during pregnancy, making it difficult to know whether a hormone level found in pregnancy is increasing or decreasing. Besides being expensive research to do, obtaining permission to study pregnant women is an exhaustive process.

Not every woman has the same amount and type of hormones. At the time of this writing, we don't really know why that is. Perhaps diet has something to do with it.

At this time, it is not known whether these hormonal situations will repeat in a subsequent pregnancy or not, or whether anything can be done to alter them. But it's important to know that there are some real biochemical differences between women who are severely sick and those who aren't. It's not all in their heads!

LEFT VERSUS RIGHT OVARY THEORY

A Swedish research team found that women whose pregnancies originated from the right ovary were significantly more affected by nausea and vomiting than women whose pregnancies originated from the left ovary. It was speculated that the progesterone produced by the corpus luteum, which surrounds the fertilized egg, may be metabolized more rapidly when produced from the left ovary. Apparently, the left ovarian vein drains into the left kidney vein, whereas the right ovarian vein drains into the inferior vena cava. The inferior vena cava is the major vein of the lower body that returns blood to the heart. Because kidneys are one of the organ systems responsible for clearing substances from the body, it's thought that they may act to reduce the hormonal load produced during pregnancy.

PROTECTION FROM SEXUAL ACTIVITY

Another theory proposes that nausea and vomiting had an evolutionary purpose: signaling to the woman's mate that she was pregnant and causing disinterest in sexual activity. This disinterest could be a mechanism to protect the developing fetus from expulsion that could result from orgasmic contractions. Although this theory doesn't speculate what causes nausea and vomiting, it might provide stress relief for a woman to know that there might be an evolutionary rationale for the suffering.

PLACENTAL ENZYMES AND LOW BLOOD SUGAR

Work in medical embryology suggests that powerful enzymes that help the fetus and placenta attach to the wall of the uterus may be responsible for the nausea and vomiting. As the placenta connects to the mother's biological system, it is said that the resulting energy drain causes low blood sugar (or hypoglycemia) in the mother, which is often reported during pregnancy. Low blood sugar has been associated with nausea, certainly in diabetes.

Despite all the brouhaha about the low blood sugar theory, there has been no study to date that can demonstrate this. The normal, healthy body provides various mechanisms to make glucose when levels are low, because glucose is the fuel needed by the brain. To make glucose, the body breaks down muscle to make sugar.

PROTECTION FROM TOXINS IN FOODS

A toxicologist from California speculates that the nausea and vomiting of pregnancy is nature's way of avoiding an accumulation of toxic substances that may originate from food, which may eventually harm the fetus. Plants and herbs contain natural chemicals that serve as herbicides. Dr. Margie Profet believes that since food stays in the stomach longer because of the influence of pregnancy hormones, the ingested food may be being evaluated for safety. If too many potential toxins are present, signals may be sent from the stomach to the brain, which in turn causes vomiting. The changing ratio of estradiol to progesterone, she feels, may be the sensing mechanism.

It may be a bit hard to accept this theory completely because if it held perfectly true, all the pregnant women who ate vegetables should be sick.

Heightened Senses

One of the major complaints I have collected in caring for hospitalized women who have debilitating morning sickness stems from a heightening of the senses. Smells can become triggers, setting off cycles of nausea and sometimes vomiting. (See Chapter 5, "Noses: Regular and Premium Odors and Morning Sickness") Other triggers are some flavors, abrupt motion, bright lights, and loud noises.

In-depth interviews with women who suffer from morning sickness provide an amazing view of the way the escalation in the sense of smell that often accompanies pregnancy can undermine the well-being of a previously healthy woman.

I believe that this enhanced sense of smell is a natural, adaptive, universal phenomenon. It might have had its beginning as a survival mechanism. As pregnancy advances, a woman's increased bulk decreases her ability to flee from danger. A sharpened sense of smell can give an advance warning of danger: smoke before a fire, ozone before a storm, or perhaps the scent of a predator on the wind.

Research indicates that one of the major pregnancy hormones, estrogen, is responsible for the increase in sensitivity to odors. It seems that the tremendous increase in estrogen itself may be proportional to this new smell threshold. Many women say that their sense of smell is greatly affected during pregnancy. Every scent is described as being heightened, more powerful, more provoking. Because most people agree that an overwhelming smell can precipitate nausea, the heightened sensitivity to smell seems to have a clear connection to the nausea.

YOUR DIET 1 YEAR BEFORE PREGNANCY

Feeling very strongly that estrogen was one of the big culprits in bad morning sickness, our group at Brigham and Women's Hospital decided to investigate the role of saturated fat from the diet and determine whether there was any association. The theory was based on the fact that saturated fat contributes to estrogen production, and estrogen is the hormone that seems to have the biggest role in the sense of smell, or olfaction. We conducted a case-controlled, matched study that paired 44 nonsick women with 44 very sick, hospitalized women according to their day of delivery. The study showed, via retrospective analysis, that the sick women had consumed higher amounts of saturated fat in their diets the year before they were pregnant. Because this was a retrospective study, we did not have blood samples of either group to see whether there were any differences in hormone levels.

PINKS VERSUS BLUES

Another theory about bad morning sickness has to do with the sex of the fetus. Do women with bad morning sickness have more estrogen because they are carrying a girl baby? It never struck me that my sick patients had girl babies than boys, because I've taken care of some pretty sick moms who have sons. Researchers have looked at fetal sex, and there are at least three recent studies that show only a slightly higher incidence of female babies and bad morning sickness. The study data suggests that 51 percent of women with bad morning sickness give birth to girls versus 49 percent who give birth to boys.

ALTERED RATIO OF T-HELPER CELLS

A research group looked at the ratio of certain types of cells called cytokines, some of which are inflammatory. The amount of the T1 cells was higher than T2 cells in pregnant women who were not sick, compared to sick women who had lower amounts of T1 cells. It is not known at this time why this occurs or if it will happen in a subsequent pregnancy. It is encouraging, however, that researchers are looking for biochemical differences in hyperemesis.

LOWER LEVELS OF B-VITAMINS

For years there has been speculation that sick women have lower levels of vitamin B_6. Certainly, in the setting of not being able to eat for days or weeks, one would expect vitamin and mineral levels to plummet. Whether being low in these vitamins before pregnancy contributes to the severity of morning sickness isn't known. It is known, however, that being in poor nutritional shape adversely affects getting pregnant in the first place!

The data about vitamin B_6 and morning sickness is variable. It was a component in one of the classic medications used to treat morning sickness: Bendectin.

Some professionals speculate that reduced levels of niacin (another B vitamin) as well as pyridoxine (vitamin B_6) may be responsible for some neurological signs and symptoms of anxiety, depression, and thought disorders that are seen in cases of malnutrition and extreme weight loss. Some think that this may also be the case with morning sickness as well. Others have mentioned that thiamine (vitamin B_1) is reduced with poor food intake and vomiting and speculate that taking in more B_1-rich foods should be helpful.

Overall, it is difficult to have a single nutrient deficiency. When you don't eat *anything*, there are about 50 nutrients missing, so a single supplement can't solve the total situation. When your stomach allows you a choice between two foods, however, it's a good idea to pick the one with the higher level of a given nutrient.

Vitamin B_6 Content of Some Foods (RDI pregnancy = 2.2 mg/day)

Food	Calories	Serving Size	mg of Vitamin B_6
Lean beef	230	3 oz	.21
Broiled cod	160	3 oz	.28
Cream of rice	240	1 cup	.07
Instant oatmeal (fortified)	100	3/4 cup	.74
Cooked spaghetti	200	1 cup	.05
Fresh strawberries	45	1 cup	.09
Cooked plantain	180	1 cup	.37
Cooked broccoli	45	1 cup	.22
Mashed potatoes w/milk	160	1 cup	.49

Vitamin B$_1$ (Thiamine) Content of Some Foods (RDI pregnancy = 1.14 mg/day)

Food	Calories	Serving Size	mg of Thiamine
Croissant	235	1	0.17
Raisin bread, enriched	65	1	0.08
Oatmeal bread, enriched	65	1	0.12
Cantaloupe melon	95	1/2	0.10
Egg	80	1	0.04
Skim milk	85	1 cup	0.09
Cooked chicken	140	3 oz	0.06
Baked potato w/skin	220	large	0.22

Chapter 4

Other Times and Other Places: Historical and Cultural Perspectives

HAZELA

Tall and stately at 5 feet, 5 inches tall and 115 pounds, this native of Trinidad experienced nausea and vomiting with all three of her pregnancies. In the late 1970s, when she was pregnant for the first time, she suffered from morning sickness for the first 4 months. During the midwinter months her weight dipped to 100 pounds. She experienced a first-trimester intolerance of milk products. A more difficult situation to manage was her excessive saliva and constant desire to spit. Her first daughter was born full-term, at 5 pounds, 8 ounces.

Two years later, Hazela was pregnant again. From day one, it was a battle to control the nausea and vomiting. Smells, perfumes, and cooking oils were all triggers for nausea, if not vomiting. Starving all day long, she often had enough appetite and desire to eat by late afternoon if her mother cooked favorite Trinidadian dishes of salted fish with boiled potatoes or salty pigtail soup.

Milk, one of her favorite foods, was again out of the question. At one point, she vomited blood and was hospitalized for dehydration for a week. Luckily, she was put in a private room. Her weight dropped 25 pounds, from 115 to 90, during the worst of the crisis. This pregnancy ended with delivery at 7 months. Weighing 3 pounds, 8 ounces, Hazela's second daughter spent 1 month in the hospital's neonatal intensive care unit and was discharged without problems.

Eight years later, the third pregnancy was punctuated by what Hazela described as "the worst case." Her prepregnancy weight was 119 pounds and dipped 10 pounds during the worst phase. Smells again were a problem. One successful remedy she discovered was Enos, an antacid from "the Islands" that she bought in her ethnic fruit store. After the morning ritual of Enos, she could keep down some soy milk, hot or cold. She could take it to work with her in a thermos. Another meal would be a soft scrambled egg made with soy milk, which she packed and ate at work with a salty sausage.

Hazela always drove her own car, saying that bus drivers would bristle if she wanted to get off at an unscheduled stop. Again, at home, whether for lunch or dinner, she was able to eat if her mother cooked. A frequent meal was highly salted fish, sauteed tomatoes with onions and green bananas, and a potato or a yam as a side dish. Another usual meal was the pigtail soup, highly salted and somewhat lumpy, with greens; ingredients included split peas, chopped potatoes, carrots, and, of course, a pig's tail.

For some unexplained reason, Hazela could cook for her household but was unable to eat what she cooked. Eating at someone else's home, however, was remarkably successful as long as the menu offered varieties of curried meat (beef, chicken, and goat), salty chicken foot soup, tripe soup, or pilah. (Pilah was described as a mixture of pigeon peas, rice, and beef or chicken.) Hazela's secret seasonings included soy sauce, garlic powder, garlic salt, hot pepper, and chili. Hazela's mother included all the same spices but added ginger and a bay leaf.

Although Hazela had read that rosemary tea was supposed to settle an upset stomach, it didn't work for her. Her beverage of choice was ice-cold grapefruit juice or sorrel tea. She brewed dried sorrel leaves, steeping them for 24 hours after sugar and clove had been added. Consumed hot or cold, sorrel tea worked.

Another successful and favorite island beverage was "Marty," made from the bark of a special tree boiled with aniseed. After it was brewed, sugar and angostura bitters were added. As it aged, it became stronger, so water was periodically added to the storage container in the refrigerator.

As with her first two pregnancies, Hazela's third and final pregnancy concluded at 7 months. Her weight, however, recovered from the low of 109 pounds to a whopping 139 pounds at delivery. Her 5-pound, 12-ounce son was hospitalized for 2 days of observation and then went home with her.

THE HISTORY OF MORNING SICKNESS TREATMENT

Morning sickness has been written about for at least 4,000 years. The first mention of nausea and vomiting during early pregnancy was found in an Egyptian papyrus scroll dating to about 2000 B.C. Hippocrates described the same symptoms in about 400 B.C. These symptoms were later referred to as *maux de coeur*, which means "sickness of the heart." The French expression, *mauvais coucheur*, or in the case of the pregnant women, *mauvaise coucheuse*, seems to describe some of the subtle manifestations of morning sickness fairly well. This phrase, which literally means a bad bedfellow or someone who is hard to live with, certainly describes any person who has the misfortune to feel waves of nausea the second she wakes up.

Modern medicine, with all its advanced equipment, antibiotics, medications, and hydration techniques, has improved health outcome dramatically in the past 50 years. Long before hydration techniques were available, most ill people were treated with medicines made from herbs or plants, which still is the basis for over 40 percent of modern medicines. This was true for the woman affected with morning sickness.

Soranus, one of the first doctors to describe this client population, had a six-step plan for treatment, heavily based on herbal concoctions.

Step 1: Women with morning sickness should not eat when they are sick. Soranus reasoned that if not eating "cured" the nausea and vomiting of seasick sailors, it might be effective in treating morning sickness.

Step 2: If a woman does eat when she is sick, she should eat easily digested foods, cold liquids, weak wine, and dry substances. Soranus also thought women should be carried in sedan chairs and should exercise both their bodies and voices to keep up their strength. (Incidentally, sedan chairs look like tiny telephone booths carried on poles, which generally sway with the motion of the carriers!)

Step 3: If the first two suggestions failed, one was to apply a mixture of freshly ground olives to the woman's abdomen and bind it with woolen bandages.

Step 4: Next, one would make the mixture of olives stronger.

Step 5: If that failed, one would add agents to this concoction: alum, aloe, saffron, pomegranate peel, oak galls, and barley meal to name a few.

Step 6: The woman was to have her extremities bound with tight bandages or be immersed in hot water.

The effectiveness of these plant-based remedies is not known. But during the Dark Ages, the use of herbs was considered pagan, so much of the experimentation was fairly secret. Monks and nuns, however, began to cultivate herbs in herb gardens, or physicks as they were called then, and there began the modern pharmacy. Herb crops were converted into potions and liquors that were dispensed to the sick and ailing.

Trotula, a woman's health-care provider who died in the year 1097 A.D. advised that women who craved to eat "potter's earth or chalk or coals" be offered "beans cooked with sugar" instead.

It is highly likely that the women described in Elisabeth Brooke's fascinating book, *Women Healers through History,* had some recipes up their sleeves for morning sickness, especially the ones who tended to women. Isis of ancient Egypt, Aspasia (of the first century) who lived in Greece, Olympias of Thebes, and Hildegard of Bingen all must have cared for women with morning sickness and had some advice. Unfortunately, finding out their secrets is not easy. In the Middle Ages many manuscripts were destroyed, and much knowledge was lost. (Of note: It may not be easy to get this book in the United States. It is published in London, and I bought it on a trip to South Africa.)

One of the earliest persons to write about herbal cures was Nicholas Culpepper, a seventeenth century astrologer-physician. For vomiting, he suggested using bilberries, bistort, buckshorn, plantain, elder, and mint. To aid digestion, he prescribed lettuce, lovage, mint, black mustard, and rosemary. Stomach ailments were treated by adding marjoram, mint, black alder, broom, and caraway. For the pregnant woman, he recommended sniffing winter savory.

A *Treatise of Midwifery*, published in England in 1781 by Alexander Hamilton, recommended that the woman with morning sickness drink camomile tea. Two years later, Charles Elliot of Edinburgh and GGJJ Robinson of London recommended rhubarb in small doses along with strengthening bitters in their book *Outline of the Theory and Practice of Midwifery*.

Aristotle's Masterpiece: or the Secrets of Nature Displayed in the Generation of Man, published in 1801, recommended several herbal remedies for women with morning sickness, including tansy syrup, mallow, violets with sugar, and common oil. Other suggestions were "avoiding disturbing passions, loud clamours, and filthy smells."

Reports from the middle 1700s give some sense of the consequences of this ailment. Kerking reported the first death in 1706. About a 100 years later, therapeutic abortion was presented as a cure for morning sickness. In 1853, the French medical society agreed with this suggestion. Ten years later, a Frenchman,

Gueniot revealed these grisly statistics: 46 of 118 women died from severe morning sickness when all his known remedies for treatment failed.

In 1855 Charlotte Bronte succumbed to morning sickness after about 11 weeks of being ill. Her slow and agonizing decline is described in Elizabeth Gaskell's biography.

In 1891, a German named Kaltenbach presented a paper before the Berlin Obstetrical Society that proclaimed that "the vomiting of pregnancy was usually a manifestation of neurosis, somewhat allied to hysteria and readily amendable to suggestive therapy."

This charge that morning sickness had a neurotic component led researchers (mostly men) to investigate every pregnant woman's psychosocial and economic backgrounds. Someone had proposed that an unmarried woman shamed by her condition of pregnancy might be more inclined to vomit. However, marital status was found to have no bearing on the incidence of morning sickness. There was also a theory, which has since been disproved, that the vomiting was a sign that the pregnancy was unwanted.

No one knows exactly what women with nausea and vomiting in early pregnancy were told by their obstetricians in the nineteenth and twentieth centuries. Because maternal mortality from morning sickness was significant, anxiety on the part of a pregnant woman might have been common. Acknowledging that even today, in the best of circumstances, nausea can be relentless, the challenges for obstetricians before the advent of modern hydration therapy must have been monumental.

Anxiety among pregnant women was undoubtedly heightened by theories about deformities in children, outlined in 1832 by French scientists Etienne and Isidore Gregory St. Hilaire.

These scientists voiced concern that hyperemesis gravidarum, the severest form of morning sickness, was the cause of some deformities.

Theoretical dialogue continued into the 1930s, 1940s, and 1950s. In 1936 a study conducted by the German scientist H. Naujoks showed that about 16 percent of the children he studied who had deformities had mothers who had been affected by hyperemesis gravidarum. In 1942 another study found that 6 of 11 mothers with vomiting in pregnancy bore deformed children, and in 1953 a scientist named Thalhammer established a relationship between vomiting in pregnancy and deformities. We now know that most women who experience mild nausea and vomiting of morning sickness have healthy babies with no deformities.

We also know that there are many environmental and genetic factors to consider when evaluating birth defects and any relationship to the nausea and vomiting of early pregnancy. But the suspected link between the reported deformities and the common occurrence of nausea and vomiting seemed to be the driving force that led many scientists, such as L. F. Hawkinson in the 1930s, to ponder the use of hormones for women with low estrogen levels in pregnancy and antiestrogens for women with high estrogen levels. In the early 1940s O. W. Smith, G. V. Smith, and S. Schiller treated women affected with morning sickness with diethylstilbesterol (DES) daily and claimed a successful, relief of nausea and vomiting in 70 percent of cases, whereas 26 percent showed improvement. DES was a drug that later was shown to be associated with a high incidence of cervical cancer in the daughters of mothers who took this drug.

The pervasive Kaltenbach theory about morning-sickness neurosis has influenced a great many clinicians for over 100 years.

H. B. Altee wrote in 1934 in the *Journal of Obstetrics and Gynecology of the British Empire* that pernicious, severe vomiting was indeed a neurotic manifestation, and he formulated a treatment program. He banned visitors to the patients for 48 hours, allowed no vomit bowl in the patient's room, allowed the patient to vomit in her bed, and instructed the nurse caring for the patient to take her time in changing the soiled linen and then feed the patient 20 minutes later. Another British researcher reported in 1945 that it was customary to send in the "most angry and foul-mouthed ward maid to clean up the mess."

One of my favorite obstetricians's found a book to share with me, *Vomiting of Pregnancy: A Symposium of the Current Literature* from 1932, published by the BiSoDol Company in New Haven, Connecticut. A night reading this tome just made my heart stop! How did women live through some of these things?

An entry by physician Franz Arzt says that free hydrochloric acid and total acid of the stomach contents are lower in pregnancy than in the nonpregnant state. This absence of free acid, he wrote, was probably a result of it being neutralized by a regurgitation of the alkaline duodenal contents into the stomach.

Another contributor, E. L. Cornell, suggested that, for best results, one should see the patient early. He also added that nasal accumulations discharging backward are not an infrequent source of vomiting.

John P. Gardiner added that, unlike other types of vomiting, morning-sickness vomiting can be elicited by stimulating the epiglottis, which is that appendage you see at the back of your throat when you open your mouth wide.

As fascinating as the theories are, the treatment section will make your eyes come out on stalks! Rectal feedings with glucose and sodium bicarbonate are suggested fairly frequently. If you had an oral diet, you'd expect to see milk, lime water, beef broth, custard, rice, and chicken. Another doctor, R. B. Howland, suggested a higher carbohydrate diet and cooked fruit, dates and raisins, green vegetables, crackers and cookies, honey, sugar, desserts, and orange and lemon juices. He suggested that the patient indulge frequently in candy, preferably the hard kind, such as fruit drops and peppermints.

One doctor, Joseph B. DeLee, was an advocate of hiding the emesis (vomit) basins. E. P. H. Harrison favored the administration of placental substance in hyperemesis gravidarum, whereas John B. Haskins recommended intravenous corpus luteum. H. D. Holman of Park Hospital Clinic at Mason City, Iowa, conducted experiments over a period of 4 years with ultraviolet irradiations.

How about this one by T. H. Jones? He used electrotherapy because it had a sedative effect! His technique consisted of placing a large, wet pad over the abdomen, the former was attached to the negative pole of a galvanic machine. Two small discs were attached to the double end of a bifurcated cord, each of which was placed over the vagus nerve in a subaural position. The single end of the cord was attached to a positive pole. The current was slowly turned on to from 15 to 20 milliamperes and maintained there for 10 minutes. This treatment was given once or twice daily, depending on how sick the woman was.

In 1939 two other theories were put forward: Karl Menninger thought that vomiting in pregnancy was caused by a "repudiation of femininity," and H. C. Hesseline believed "the vomiting was a form of self-punishment." In the same year, Menninger also wrote that the type of person most affected by hyperemesis was "well to do" or the intellectual college girl. He argued that the syndrome was not prevalent in Southern black women or the poor and uneducated. G. Gladstone Robertson, writing in 1946 in England's influential *Lancet* said that a high proportion of the women who suffered from nausea and vomiting in pregnancy were, at the times of their marriages, overly attached to their mothers and had some degree of sexual revulsion toward their husbands. He did not study the degree of maternal attachment or sexual revulsion outside the context of nausea and vomiting of pregnancy. Robertson noted that one-third of these women continued to be sick beyond the fifth month of pregnancy, whereas the majority two-thirds were sick 6 weeks or fewer.

In the early 1960s, Denys Fairweather from London used a health questionnaire, the Cornell Medical Index, along with the Minnesota Multiphasic Personality Inventory to conclude that these 44 women had a "marked association with a hysterical personality." Fairweather went on to say that there was little doubt that psychiatric factors must be implicated in 75 to 80 percent of the cases of severe morning sickness.

MORNING SICKNESS AND FOOD CRAVINGS AROUND THE WORLD

It is difficult to know the worldwide incidence of morning sickness, because the incidences are not recorded. According to a source at the Office of International Statistics located in Hyattsville, Maryland, their office does not yet cover health codes past 469. Hyperemesis gravidarum, the most extreme case of morning sickness, has an International Classification of Disease (ICD) code of 643. The ICD codes are a series of numbers that describe various disease or health conditions in all countries. These codes are a way to trace the prevalence of health problems. In the United States our system is fairly well developed, and the use of computers has made it easier to send data from hospitals and health-care centers to a central data collection.

Despite the lack of statistical information for the international incidence of morning sickness, it is highly unlikely that morning sickness does not exist worldwide. In my interviews with tribal women in South Africa I learned many things about the way their culture treats morning sickness. For example, most health problems are treated at the tribal level, and the Xhosa women affected by nausea and vomiting of pregnancy are given bark water to drink. Contrarily, the Zulu women may eat a few balls of bland clay or chalk daily until the nausea and vomiting abate. Indian women in the South African region are reported to eat the sour tamarind fruit. There is evidence in the botanical literature of active ingredients in rosemary, thyme, sweet fennel, horehound, anise, and cumin that account for their use in treating morning sickness in other cultures.

Clay and chalk balls each have different properties, depending on the region of the world where they were collected and their color. For example, the red clay from Mississippi may have a high content of iron as well as aluminum, whereas gray-colored clay from Georgia may have little iron but substantially more aluminum. (Of note: Soil can be contaminated by parasites and industrial wastes.) A. R. P. Walker and colleagues from a prestigious South African university and research institute found that a high percentage of black women who ate clay reported less severe nausea and vomiting associated with pregnancy. Unfortunately, the type of clay or earth eaten was not described. However, it was noted that the mixed-race women ate soil and ice, the Indian women ingested soil and clay (though in lesser amounts), and the white women consumed some chalk and ice.

The field work of some notable geographers and anthropologists, such as John Hunter, Donald Vermeer, and Miles Richardson, points to some new dimensions of earth eating, especially in cultural groups. Vermeer found, for example, that the clays eaten ritually are composed primarily of potassium and calcium. Ghanian women also have a superstition about not swallowing saliva, thinking that it makes them sicker. Women in the United States who have excessive saliva report the same thing.

Some clay has been reported to have properties that resemble those of milk of magnesia. Thanks to its absorptive and neutralizing makeup, the use of activated charcoal was used for the treatment of gastric ulcers and other gastrointestinal ailments in the 1920s. Medical reports can be found in such prestigious journals as *The Lancet*, the *Canadian Medical Journal*, and the *Hahnemannian Monthly*.

There are cultural and religious attachments to geophagy, or the eating of earth, as noted by the team of geographers lead by John Hunter in 1989 as well as by Miles Richardson and William Davidson as they visited the community of Esquipulas, Guatemala. Here clay is molded into religious figures called *panito del señor* and blessed in the Shrine of the Black Christ, or *el Christo Negro*. This special clay is considered "cool" and is thought to relieve the discomforts of pregnancy, which are considered "hot." Clay of this region is of the smectite variety and contains calcium, which is easily stripped out, expands in fluid and is thought to reduce gastric acidity. Georgia clay, as I noted before, is lower in iron; white or gray clays are higher in other minerals. Clay eating has been reported to reduce excessive salivation as well as altered taste and smell.

Anemia in pregnancy may be worsened by eating clay because it may reduce gastric acid secretions by absorption. A certain amount of gastric acid is needed to turn ferric iron into ferrous iron, the form the body uses to prevent anemia. This is not to say that I am suggesting you run out and eat clay! There are real concerns that eating clay can also deliver you a case of parasites or some nasty environmental toxins, because one never knows where hazardous wastes are disposed. There are case reports of various soil parasites being imbedded in brain tissue.

Likewise, eating cornstarch, a dry, bland, odorless, and smooth source of calories, has been implicated in promoting iron-deficiency anemia, probably because it contains no nutrients except for calories. Some women find that eating a tablespoon of cornstarch does the trick to reduce nausea. Cornstarch is a food substance. Some women can eat a box at a time, which can contribute a hefty amount of calories.

Treatments for morning sickness in other cultures range from the use of herbal teas to the eating of dry clay or chalk-like substances. One woman from Barbados said she knew many women who would eat dry arrowroot starch and travel miles into the country to get a special clay. Our woman Hazela, from Trinidad, said that Enos, a relative of Alka-Selzter, was a popular treatment in her area. Another Caribbean woman said that some women would travel to a remote but pristine sparkling beach to drink sea water. An Indian woman remarked that her friends would simmer a blend of spices, predominantly anise, and drink the elixir. Some would take it hot, others ice cold.

Eating nonnutritive substances is different by culture. In a study of 160 women enrolled in the WIC program in Long Beach, California, four researchers found that a small number from each of four ethnic groups craved and ate items considered abnormal for their culture.

In the group of black women, 2 percent ate clay, 5 percent ingested laundry starch, 3 percent ate paper, and no one ate plaster. In the Cambodian group, there were no clay eaters, but 5 percent ate laundry starch, 7 percent paper, and 7 percent plaster. Among the white women, 5 percent ate laundry starch only, and in the Hispanic group, 2 percent ate paper only. We have no idea why. Eating these substances is a concern because chemicals and toxic agents can be found in all categories.

When I find women who eat unusual substances, I try to find the closest relative that is harmless. For example, someone eating laundry starch could be eating either the crunchy type or the smooth and soft type. Once I figure out this first characteristic, I try to match up something safe. If it's the crunchy type, for example, maybe potato sticks would be okay. If it is the smooth type, maybe I'd offer cornstarch. I would also check to see whether the woman had M.S.S., or mega saliva syndrome, going on. Maybe it's a chronic nausea issue that could be reduced by eating the substance being craved (or one similar to it); maybe it's a generational pregnancy "gotta do this" bit of advice. Also, look at what other ethnic relatives have tried and know what's in the background already. This is where the spice world can open up.

Ginger has been used in several cultures to quell nausea. In most hospitals, ginger ale is a preferred beverage for nauseated patients. Eating solid ginger, such as baker's cut ginger pieces, is also a way to get ginger, and don't forget about ginger jam on your toast. Or you can use powdered ginger mixed with sugar and sprinkled on hot cream of wheat.

Eating lemons has been noted as a remedy for seasickness. In my clinical experience, lemons have a real therapeutic effect, but only if a woman has never gotten sick on them before. Patients can do whatever they wish with their fresh lemons. Some sniff them, others suck wedges plain, and some eat them sprinkled with salt. It is true that lemons are acidic and that repeatedly eating them may harm dental enamel, but so will vomiting, and the lemon therapy never lasts long. Lemon also contains vitamin C, an antioxidant that everyone needs.

I've also found that cinnamon seems to work to reduce nausea. Remember those round red "Fireball" candies we ate as kids? I've given those out in the hospital and, for some women, sucking on them helps. It certainly distracts them from the saliva issue, which we'll get to shortly. I've also given out cinnamon sticks and had women use them in hot tea. You can always add cinnamon sugar to your toast or oatmeal.

Then there is ice eating, or pagophagia. Interestingly, this has been associated with iron-deficiency anemia, but women who eat ice for hydration are generally eating very few high-nutrient foods, simply because of nausea and vomiting. Many women are often slightly anemic before pregnancy and are unaware of it until they begin seeing a doctor on a regular basis. A common reason for anemia is heavy monthly blood losses before pregnancy combined with marginal diets. So once a woman has morning sickness and sees her doctor, her anemia may have gotten worse. Whether one can blame eating ice on the anemia in pregnancy is questionable. Ice and water provide few nutrients but are vital to sustaining metabolic processes. One of my clients said the ice was the only thing that could reduce the feeling of fire in the back of her throat, the result of endless vomiting episodes.

Besides eating different cultural bandage foods, women in less-developed countries are often more closely tied to a network of other women. When one member is unable to perform her usual duties, most of the others divide up and perform her tasks as a matter of course. Unfortunately, this sort of selfless camaraderie is generally lacking in highly sophisticated countries today.

CULTURAL PREFERENCES FOR FOOD

Hazela's food preferences are unique to her culture, although they might be somewhat unusual for the typical yuppie's palate. Researchers have looked at which foods various groups of women crave and avoid in pregnancy. Of course, one can not assume that *all* women in a cultural group will follow these observations, but the results of the research in this section will help you appreciate why it's a challenge for physicians and care providers to try to make a "one size fits all" diet for pregnant women.

The facts of the study are these: Four ethnic groups—blacks, Cambodians, whites, and Hispanic—of pregnant women all had different food-group cravings one or more times per week. The order of preferences is different and fascinating:

Black women: apples, melons, avocados, mangoes, papayas.

Cambodian women: apples, mangoes, papayas, and melons and avocados were tied even.

White women: apples, melons, avocados and mangoes. There were no cravings for papayas.

Hispanic women: apples, avocados, melons, mangoes, and papayas.

This study does not specify whether the preferred apples were red or green, both of which have difference tastes and textures. I would bet that green apples would be Grannie Smith's, but that's just a guess.

When we get to pigs' feet, more craving were reported among Cambodian women (52 percent), followed by Hispanic women (32 percent), black women (12 percent), and white women (10 percent).

By the way, before you say anything about animals' feet—other than "yuck!"—you should read what was recommended in the United States from the *Practical Cooking and Serving* cookbook, fashionable in 1921. (Just read a few more pages!)

Cheese had a high rating for cravings: 87 percent among Hispanic women, to a low of 62 percent in Cambodian women. Pickles were another item that carried high marks: 55 percent for Cambodian women and 62 percent for the other groups. If I were to guess, because this study did not provide data, I would say that dill pickles were craved more often than sweet pickles. I suspect that each of these cultures would undoubtedly have their own pickle recipe. I can say that with a serious degree of certainty, because I collect ethnic cookbooks and have probably 50 of them.

Fermented fish was craved by about 50 percent of Cambodian and Hispanic women, dropping to half of that by black and white women.

Preference for tofu really surprised me: 97 percent of Hispanic women craved it, then 60 percent of Cambodian women, followed by black and white women at 3 percent and 2 percent, respectively.

Food aversions also have a curious distribution. Ice cream was adverse to 15 percent of Cambodian women, 5 percent of black women, 3 percent of Hispanic women, and 0 percent of white women.

Cactus also had a curious distribution of aversion: 68 percent of black women found it aversive, 48 percent of white women, 38 percent of Cambodian women, and 35 percent of Hispanic women. But, I'm sure it depends on how long you have lived where this food grows and what your neighbors eat.

Basically, there is no predicting what pregnant women will want to eat at all! Remember that game the *64,000-Dollar Question* (which is really pocket change these days to many)? Well, these questions could be part of the game show and would probably always be a mystery!

FEEDING THE INVALID: THE HISTORY OF MORNING SICKNESS MANAGEMENT

Becoming interested in the history of morning sickness and hyperemesis management has been a very worthwhile self-education. Effective morning sickness and hypermesis management seems to revolve around culinary anf herbal finesse, positive mind-body work, appreciation of olfactory enhancement, and hydration intervention.

Regarding food for really sick people, one book in particular, *Ouma's Cookery*, which I bought in South Africa at the Colonel Smuts historic home in Irene, is an eye opener. Colonel Smuts not only was the organizer of the League of Nations after World War I but also an incredible botanist in his own right, with an amazing collection of species preserved by one person with a serious dedication to the art and science. The tour of his home and property was outstanding on all fronts—even on a 90°F day.

Smuts's wife, Ouma, penned a cookbook, which the local historical society republished. It is a tourist thing to buy; so, of course, I bought one. In the 1940s, cookbooks from the UK had sections on feeding the invalid. That was the trend in those days.

Ouma provided suggestions of what foods to try. Although these are not earmarked for morning sickness, it's worth thinking through these two recipes and why or how they work, if they do.

Rice Water (from Ouma)

Wash 2 ounces of rice well, then sprinkle into 4 pints boiling water. Add a small piece of lemon rind and allow to cook for half an hour. Strain and sweeten to taste and leave in a cool place. (For a food safety point, I'd suggest drinking it immediately or putting it in the refrigerator and trying it cold)

Invalid Jelly (from Ouma)

1/2 oz gelatine, 1/2 pt water, 1/4 pt orange juice, 2 eggs, 1/2 cup sugar, lemon rind

Place sugar, gelatine, water, and rind of one small lemon in a sauce pan. Stir until the gelatin dissolves, then add orange juice and bring to a boil. Cool the mixture and pour over beaten eggs, stirring all the time. Strain and pour into a wet mould.

Ouma has other interesting recipes. You can probably buy her cookbook online if you are interested.

The bottom line is that if a particular food or dish feels like it will work, find someone to make it for you pronto! Friends need recipes so that if they are trying to help you, they can do it the right way—as best they can. If you have favorite comfort food recipes, try to dig them out. They can be useful. If you hire a personal chef to help out, they too would need a recipe.

Flaxseed Tea from *Practical Cooking and Serving* is fascinating! Again, it is for invalids—in this case, women who have severe morning sickness.

Flaxseed Tea

Blanch 2 tablespoons of flaxseeds; take 1 quart of boiling water and let boil 1 to 2 hours; strain and add lemon juice and sugar. (You have to wonder, if the water evaporates, should you add more? This probably wouldn't be a consideration these days, because most folks today wouldn't spend 10 minutes in the kitchen, let alone 1 hour!)

Practical Cooking and Serving also suggests the following:
Peptonized milk
Almond milk soup
Lemon, vinegar, or wine whey
Beef tea custard
Egg and wine
Wheat flour and cornmeal gruel
Irish moss lemonade
Toast water or bread tea
Currant and tamarind water
Calf's foot jelly

The *Rumford Cookbook,* on the other hand, suggests albumenized milk. This is made with 1 egg white, 1/4 cup lime water, and 1 cup milk. You put it in a shaker, shake it, strain it, and serve it plain or with sugar. (Obviously, today, the raw egg could be considered a food-safety issue.)

The *Rumford Cookbook* also suggests making and serving the sickly person a mixture of lemonade, barley water, toast water, eggnog, wine whey (which is milk flavored with 2 tablespoons of commercial sherry flavoring), acid phosphate whey, beef and tapioca broth, and "Invalid's Tea" (which is 1 level teaspoon of plain tea, 1 cup of scalded milk, and sugar to taste). They use loose tea and strain the concoction before serving. Gruels were popular— cornmeal, arrowroot, oatmeal, name your cereal! Irish moss is on the menu. One final suggestion is scraped beef sandwiches. Take lean steak from which you remove all the fat, cut the meat into strips, scrape the pulp from the fiber, and season. Spread this on thin slices of bread or toast, buttered or plain, and serve. They don't say whether the meat is cooked or raw, so it's anyone's guess!

I'll have to try the dyspeptic bread. This bread is to be eaten by those who have a weak digestive system and who cannot assimilate bread prepared with yeast. The recipe calls for 1 pint flour, 1 teaspoon salt, 4 teaspoons baking powder, and milk or water to mix. No amounts are given for liquids. This should make for an interesting morning in the kitchen!

MEDICINAL FOODS AND RECIPES FROM AROUND THE WORLD

While perusing the cookbook *Indian Delights*, which I bought in South Africa, I was delighted to find a section in the back titled "Convalescence and Remedial Foods." Although some of the ingredients are not known to me, this cookbook's author notes some practical remedies. Ginger Paak is a remedy for colds that also contains ground almonds and coconut. There's a Poppy Seed Milk recipe for insomnia and headache, a recommendation that Methi (mint) water should be consumed before breakfast, and an emphasis on fresh juices. The Masala Tea recipe includes a few ingredients I do not know, but I do recognize some of its ingredients: dry ginger, cinnamon, and cloves.

The *Chinese System of Food Cures*, by Henry C. Lu, suggests dried mandarin orange peel for vomiting and lack of appetite, red or green pepper for vomiting, peppermint for indigestion, radish for vomiting, tomato for poor appetite, button mushrooms for vomiting, white rice for morning sickness, chicken for poor appetite, cuttlefish for excessive gastric acid, and vinegar for vomiting of blood. For herbs and spices, Lu recommends star anise for vomiting, fennel seed for vomiting, sweet basil for indigestion, cinnamon bark for abdominal pain, dillseed for poor appetite, cloves for abdominal pain, ginger for vomiting and the common cold, nutmeg and marjoram for vomiting, Chinese parsley (coriander) for indigestion, and black and white pepper for upset stomach and vomiting of clear water.

Apples are recommended for morning sickness. Coconut is recommended for vomiting, grapefruit for poor appetite in pregnant women, lemon for indigestion, tangerine for vomiting, and pineapple for vomiting. The book also suggests boiling 15 to 20 grams of grapefruit peel in water and drinking the tea to relieve morning sickness.

Here is another recipe to relieve morning sickness: Fry 250 grams of sweet rice with 30 milliliters of fresh ginger juice until the rice breaks, then grind it into a powder. Take 10 to 20 grams in warm water each time, twice a day, until you are better.

There is a recipe that calls for boiling 60 milliliters of rice vinegar, to which you add 30 grams of sugar and stir until dissolved. Then you break an egg into this mixture and cook it. When the egg is done, you drink the whole thing. I believe that you probably scramble the egg before you put it in the rice-sugar solution, but the book doesn't say.

Here is one final recipe from that book: Steam 9 grams of grapefruit peel and 12 grams of Chinese salted brown olives in 600 to 700 milliliters of water until the olives are fully cooked. After taking this five to seven times, it's supposed to cure morning sickness!

Chapter 5

Noses: Regular and Premium Odors and Morning Sickness

GRETA

Tall, attractive, athletic, and professionally accomplished would describe the strawberry blonde, Scandinavian-looking Greta. When she was admitted for care in the early weeks of her first—and only—pregnancy she reported comments others had made to her; some of which she found insensitive. She was a research cardiac program director with many nutrition courses under her belt. Some of her first-time-mother friends, nonpregnant colleagues, and immediate family asked her point blank why she couldn't eat better and take care of herself well enough to avoid hospitalization, given her extensive personal knowledge about nutrition.

Greta wasn't sure what variety of morning sickness she might be having. Was she way beyond the garden variety of morning sickness? Had she graduated to hyperemesis gravidarum and she didn't know? There were no set guidelines she could find. Because Greta was also an athlete, she was worried about her bone health. A few years before, she'd fractured a bone in her foot during an intense marathon. She made it a point to keep her calcium intake optimal. However, once the morning sickness started, dairy products were out the window.

When Greta was hospitalized for the first setback, we explored the role of various smells that disturbed her state of well-being. Greta thought of certain odors at home that sent her over the edge. The smell of cooking pasta, she could say with certainty, was a problem. Her husband's specialty was pasta—prepared in at least 100 varieties! No longer able to practice his culinary talents at home, the solution was for him to cook the pasta at his mother's house and bring it home to heat in a microwave.

Greta returned to work part-time after her first hospitalization but was only 50 percent efficient. Doodling one day at her desk, Greta came up with an acronym for her nose. She joked that her nose was a "capital nose." Nose became N.O.S.E.S., for neonatal observatory for safe environmental situations.

She envisioned her developing baby sending messages to hightail it whenever local air-borne pollutant levels became extreme. She would heed the early clues of N.O.S.E. whenever she could. She figured if she blamed it on the baby, people might pay more attention to her complaints.

Greta found a quote she absolutely treasured, "All genius is in my nostrils" was quoted from Freidrich Nietzsche in *Scent: The Mysterious and Essential Powers of Smell*, a book given to her years previously as a birthday gift.

Another new problem was the devoted family dog, Maxwell (Max, for short). Suddenly Max smelled more "doggy" to Greta. This overly friendly St. Bernard–Basset hound hybrid, a pup from the rescue shelter, matured into a 3-year-old devoted 80-pound walking companion. At 5 a.m. he would trot beside Greta for her daily early morning exercise regime.

Now, he'd follow Greta to the bathroom, often keeping her company during bouts of vomiting. His antics of licking her toes now became a total nuisance. The St. Bernard part of his genetics produced the typical drooling habit, which became a sight that would add to Greta's misery.

Greta thought "now we are both drooling! I *hate* mine and I *hate his!*" The drooling was bad enough, but the dog's breath was beyond description.

Yelling at the dog produced 80 pounds of canine meltdown. Face between paws and quietly and intermittently whimpering, Max hadn't done anything criminal: he was a just a dog in the wrong place at the wrong time.

To Greta's husband, Rick, the dog smelled no different now than ever before, and he was upset that the immediate solution meant Greta and the dog couldn't be in the same room. The dog was a present from Greta to Rick on his thirtieth birthday—something both of them talked long and hard about once they saw those big brown saucer eyes staring from the other side of a steel grate. And if Max could talk, he would always say, "Thanks for adopting me!" His size intimidated most strangers, even though he never growled or bared his fangs. He was never more than 2 feet from Greta and Rick—no leash was ever required on a beach or neighborhood walks. Other dogs never upset him. He was Mr. Canine Mellow. Everyone knew it.

Rick loved his dog, but he now learned that any doggie drool had to be mopped up immediately, or more disastrous events would happen. Greta had secret thoughts from time to time of giving the dog Sominex so he'd sleep through her pregnancy. Sometimes she had more permanent thoughts about the dog and would feel horribly that she wished unkind events to an always kind, in your face, and loving pet that she had happily walked with at 5 a.m. for months before this pregnancy happened.

Five feet, eight inches tall, Greta started her pregnancy at 115 pounds and hit a low of 98 pounds when she was hospitalized for a second time. Her weight dropped by 17 pounds, and she was malnourished. Greta's doctors sent her for an endoscopy to rule out an ulcer, because some of her emesis was blood-tinged.

The endoscopy required that a small tube be inserted down Greta's throat, which was anesthetized with a xylocaine spray. Through the tube, the radiologist could view the interior of Greta's stomach, which showed some tears—Mallory-Weiss tears. These were not uncommon to find when anyone has had an extensive course of vomiting, she was told. As Greta feared, she gagged through a good part of the examination; her gag point was definitely lower. Luckily, her nausea did not escalate into vomiting. A test for H. *pylori* turned out to be negative. H. *pylori*, Greta was told, was a common bad bug for some folks with gastro-intestinal problems and had been found in some cases of bad morning sickness (see the appendix for more on H. *pylori*).

Hospitalized for 5 days and then home for another 3 1/2 weeks, Greta returned to work part-time. She would drive into the city after rush hour to minimize the likelihood of getting behind a garbage truck or bus. She avoided bumpy roads and sudden stops. When her husband drove, Greta had to remind him that bumps and jolts might be trigger factors and to drive at an even speed, avoiding quick curves and abrupt stops. Rick, thinking himself the Mario Andretti of Route 128 in Boston, hated driving his Corvette as slowly as Greta drove their station wagon. "Hey Mario, the dreadful driver," Greta would say, "*Please* watch the bumps and twists! Or your seats will find out what I had for breakfast!" Greta was anything but pleased when her husband would get a mild case of road rage on the commute to work.

She brought lunch to work: marshmallow rice squares, baked potatoes, and vanilla yogurt. She also brought a bag filled with lemon wedges. Her lunch was a far cry from her former choices of whole-wheat pita, skim milk, and vegetarian salad with chickpeas and tofu cheese. Greta would sniff lemons most of the day and would add several to glasses of bottled water.

During the pregnancy, Greta kept a diary of events and noted comments made by well-meaning friends and relatives while she was sick. Two of the most irritating comments were "Just use positive thinking, it'll go away" and "Oh, you have to eat something." A friend took Rick aside and offered this advice: "You just have to be ruthless and make her eat!" Greta reflected, "When you're nauseous half the time and vomiting the other half, the last thing you care to read about is the basic food groups and how eating a few crackers will fix you right up!"

After 23 weeks, Greta started to feel normal again and began to gain weight. Because she spent a lot of time being a couch potato, her muscles felt like jelly. She wondered how she used to jog! At 40 weeks her weight was up to 130 pounds, for a gain of 32 pounds from her lowest weight. Despite more speculations that the baby had to be a girl because she was so sick, Greta delivered, via cesarean section, an 8-pound, 4-ounce baby boy.

THE RADAR NOSE OF PREGNANCY

Years ago I coined the phrase *radar nose of pregnancy* as a shortcut for a bigger term of *hyperolfaction* (which basically means super-smeller). Sick women knew exactly what the term meant without a lot of explanation. They were living with radar noses 24/7. (Maybe a better term would be *hyperolfaction emesis*—meaning "super smells create vomiting.")

Smells have a lot to do with morning sickness. Smells are invisible, so it is difficult to put a fence around them. What you won't easily know is whether people you know suffer from hyposmia (pronounced "hi-poz-me-a") or a diminished sense of smell. If someone doesn't have a great sense of smell, sometimes they don't know it because they've lived with it for a long time, and they have no reference. Dr. Susan Schiffman reported that about 2 million American adults had disorders of taste and smell in 1983. This figure is likely much higher because some people just decide to live with it.

The fact that many people have a poor sense of smell can make it difficult to control smells from people, places, and circumstances. Locations can have subtle odor changes during a 24-hour period.

Take the bedroom, for example. If you sleep with the bedroom windows closed, the air will smell quite stale by morning. A woman with morning sickness will notice it, whereas her spouse might not. It seems also the smaller the room, the staler the air. Bedroom air may be adverse in the morning if the bedroom is too close to a kitchen, bathroom, or the bedroom of an incontinent elderly person or young child. The air in your bedroom may also smell bad if it is on the street side and local garbage collection is a regular occurrence, with one of those monster stink-mobiles (Yuck! Even for a nonpregnant nose).

Most know that morning breath, also known as dog breath, can be fierce, and you may be able to smell what your bed partner ate the night before because of breath vapors. A sleeping body gives off fumes at night, either by exhaling or in perspiration. Strong-smelling foods and beverages, such as garlic, onions, broccoli, pepperoni sausages, and beer tend to make their presence known—residual fragrances also come through body pores.

Clinical practice has convinced me that most of the physical complaints of morning sickness begin with the nose, thanks to the influence of pregnancy hormones. As women examine the role of odors in triggering the nausea and vomiting of morning sickness, they'll have more control of their own well-being.

A researcher from Halifax, Nova Scotia, looked at pregnant women's senses of smell by each trimester and pregnancy and validated that the first trimester is where the heightened senses are most likely.

The function of the nose is to filter and warm air with each breath. For the developing fetus as well as the mother, oxygen (transferred by the lungs to the blood) is needed to properly metabolize food. In the course of metabolism, the waste products of carbon dioxide are exhaled through the mouth and nose.

During pregnancy a woman takes in more breaths per minute. One hormone that is believed to be responsible for increasing the respiration rate is estrogen. Estrogen is also thought to enhance the sense of smell. Nausea, too, is said to increase sensitivity to odors. Although an enhanced sense of smell is really a benefit (it can protect you and your baby against dangers ranging from spoiled food to fire), the drawback is nausea.

Let's face it—smells are ubiquitous. They're connected with people; they lurk in your household and workplace; they're part of the outdoors. Once you've figured out which smells trigger the nausea of morning sickness, you may or may not be able to take evasive actions. Everyone in your office will probably agree that the city garbage heap half a mile away means the windows can't be opened when the wind is blowing from that direction. However, everyone may not agree that the smell of gourmet coffee cooking away all morning in the pot constitutes a major health hazard (even though the oils from coffee *do* turn rancid with prolonged heat and change into unhealthy substances that are not good for you).

Some smells that tend to trigger morning sickness are more obvious than others. Women who live in large housing complexes complain about the cooking smells from each apartment both in winter, when closed windows keep in the odors, and in summer, when heat and humidity trap food smells in hallways. For some of the women I have counseled, the only solution is to find another living situation for a while. Some smells are more subtle triggers, such as the odor of stale cardboard boxes in kitchen cupboards. For the most part, trigger smells are very ordinary and are ignored by the average nonpregnant person.

The "Where the Smells Are" section lists some sources of odors that are troublesome for women with morning sickness. Read them over and also make your own list of bad trigger smells. As you'll find out, the world is made up of many good smells and bad smells.

LET'S HEAR IT FOR LEMONS!

For years, we've been giving out lemons for our morning-sickness patients to sniff or lick. Lemon is a fragrance that works about 99 percent of the time. I've never really been able to explain why lemon works, but there is some new research about lemons and health improvement. Dr. Theodore Postolache at the National Institute of Mental Health has been exploring the role of various smells on depression, seasonal affective disorder, and mood. Although he has not studied morning-sickness women, his outstanding work supports the role of lemon fragrance in well-being.

WHERE THE SMELLS ARE

THE HEAD

Your hair needs to be shampooed regularly, because it produces oils that can trap odors from food and smoke. Some hairstyles, such as once-a-week French twists and cornrows, may not be the best idea at this time, because they're shampooed less often. Shampoos, cream rinses and conditioners, hair sprays, and home permanents also contribute perfume smells.

THE FACE

Aftershave and men's colognes often top the trigger list. Moisturizing lotions and makeup can also set off bouts of nausea. Besides perfume scents in aftershaves and colognes, expect most brands to contain phlytates, a chemical compound that has been shown to have health adversities.

THE MOUTH

Everybody's breath has some odor, and depending on what you or your companions have eaten and your general physical health and oral hygiene, breath can seem unusually powerful to you when you're coping with morning sickness. Alcohol, coffee, and cigarettes on the breath are generally considered the worst. Dentures can emit odors, too.

Worried about being rude or insensitive, many pregnant women learn to simply hold their breath. But if the smell of your family's or friends' breath is causing episodes of nausea and vomiting, you need to find a way to discuss the problem, perhaps by sharing this book.

THE HANDS

Some chemical and food smells seem to become permanently embedded in skin. A cook who chops onions and garlic all day can attest to this, as can a mechanic whose hands smell of grease. Rubbing the hands and fingers with lemon juice eliminates strong food odors; a gritty hand-soap powder helps get rid of grease smells, or if its smell doesn't bother you, Avon Skin-So-Soft works well, too.

UNDERARMS

Besides the number-one problem of poor hygiene, the perfumes added to deodorants sometimes add insult to injury. A new unscented deodorant may help. Or maybe changing the soap in the bathtub to a menthol-smelling, tea tree soap.

FEET

Shoes can become moldy and musty. Synthetic linings in inexpensive shoes and sneakers are more likely to make feet hot and sweaty. Some people take their shoes off under their desks, but for the pregnant woman, out of sight is not out of mind. If the person whose feet or shoes bother you is a family member, suggest deodorant insoles. Dirty, damp, and smelly socks sometimes lurk under a bed or other bedroom furniture. Get them into the wash immediately. More frequent or thorough foot washing or the use of foot powder may help. Sprinkling in a few tablespoons of baking soda overnight and then vacuuming the shoes out might cut down on bad shoe smell.

CLOTHING

Wash clothes promptly after wearing them. Remember that clothes worn when cooking or where people are smoking pick up these odors. Some dirty cleaners cut costs by not changing their cleaning fluids regularly; if your clothes don't come back smelling quite clean, mention it to the cleaner.

THE KITCHEN

Kitchen curtains hold cooking odors and should be washed frequently in mild soap. Over time, kitchen walls also collect a thin film of grease from cooking. To create a relatively aroma-free kitchen, have someone sponge down all surfaces, including the ceiling. Be sure that the cleansing solution is fairly diluted and has no added perfume; you don't want to replace one odor with another that may be just as offensive. Baking soda and warm water make a neutralizing rinse after a thorough wipe-down. To wash her kitchen floor, one of my clients added several fresh, cut-up lemons to a bucket of warm water.

Your tap water may smell funny to you, although that doesn't necessarily mean there's anything wrong with it. If the odor bothers you, try a filtered water container before you start to invest in bottled water. Try to keep your exposure to plastic containers to a minimum. Plastic containers are not as inert as glass containers. Add lemon slices!

Many stores now offer customers a choice between paper and biodegradable plastic bags. Some of the biodegradable bags smell like burnt rubber, which may provide another irritant.

Check the pans under your stove burners for food spills. Ovens overdue for cleaning can emit rancid grease smells, especially when the heat is on.

Keep the refrigerator clean. (Someone other than you, of course!) Toss out any leftovers more than 2 days old. Not only do leftovers lose their flavor and some nutritional value, but dangerous bacteria begin to accumulate. Pregnancy reduces immune function, so pregnant women are more susceptible to food poisoning than nonpregnant women.

If possible, have someone else clean the inside of the refrigerator and wash and dry all the trays and drawers thoroughly. Don't forget the freezer. Even if your freezer is frost-free, you may find nearly prehistoric food in the far corners. Check for any poorly wrapped foods, because they can impart flavors to the ice cubes. Once the freezer and refrigerator are clean, put a new box of baking soda in both and extra boxes in the vegetable bins to absorb odor. Date the boxes and change them every few months. In between changes, shake up the contents so that a new layer of baking soda is on top. Use the old baking soda in water as a rinse to freshen up the shower or bathtub or to sprinkle down the kitchen and bathroom drains.

There's likely to be some smelly stuff in the kitchen drain. Instead of pouring corrosive chemicals down the pipes, a handy person might try wiggling a wire around to loosen any mysterious mass, which can then be flushed away with a generous stream of water, and that "handy person" cannot be you! Some under-the-sink traps are easy to clean: Just unscrew the large nut at the bottom. A few tablespoons of baking soda in the drain will freshen it up a bit. If you have a smelly garbage disposal, check the equipment manual for suggestions on cleaning and preventive maintenance. Run some lemon rinds through the disposal. Don't forget to have someone check the dishwasher for hidden pieces of food chunks around the drain. Never stick your hand in the garbage disposal!

THE BATHROOM

What goes for kitchen drains holds true for bathroom drains. Wipe down the tiles in the shower or tub with a mild detergent. (Never use bleach and ammonia together; the combination can produce deadly fumes.) Wipe surfaces instead of spraying; sprays send extra chemicals into the air. Read labels and try to find a cleaner without propellants or perfumes, or use baking soda dissolved in water. Keep the shower curtain clean, too; wipe both sides with a fungicide and dry them thoroughly. If the curtain is machine washable, wash it. Hang the curtain outside in the sun for a while if possible: The sun's ultraviolet rays will help kill any lingering mildew. Consider buying a new curtain or an inexpensive liner.

You may want to avoid highly scented soaps. The hot water of a shower vaporizes the perfume in soaps. Soaps with natural orange, lemon, green apple, or cinnamon scents may be more refreshing. Discard or give away any perfumed bath cubes that may be hanging around your bathroom.

THE BEDROOM

Household aromas can creep into your room at any time. A draft dodger, one of those long fabric tubes, can keep smells from coming in under the door. Draft dodgers are easy to make and are also available in many mail-order catalogs.

Laundry detergents and fabric softeners can impart strong fragrances to nightclothes and bedding and can disturb your sleep. Try switching to an unscented detergent and softener. If you have to sleep away from home, take along your own pillow or take two pillowcases to cut down on the odor of a strange pillow. Another defensive strategy is to put a favorite herbal tea bag inside a pillowcase. Use a familiar, mildly scented tea, such as mint or lemon; use a favorite hard candy, such as cherry; or use a more pungent familiar smell, such as that of a cough drop.

THE WORKPLACE

The main complaint of pregnant women may well be the collective coffeepots. Office coffeepots are notorious for sitting around all day and releasing the smell of scorched coffee, which by 11:15 a.m. is pretty much indistinguishable from the aroma of burning tires. I know that I am repeating myself with the coffee business, but this is deliberate. I cannot make this point strongly enough. There are at least 62 volatile compounds that start to form and change with the heat of brewing coffee.

Workplace rest rooms are often not vented to the outside, and most have air fresheners in them that give off a fragrance designed to be stronger than the bathroom odors.

Many office buildings (and homes) are poorly ventilated in general, and more and more synthetic materials are being used for carpets, cabinets, countertops, and the like that give off chemical odors that may be particularly irksome to pregnant women, as well as probably hazardous to other employees' health.

DO ANIMALS GET MORNING SICKNESS?

The question of whether or not animals get morning sickness is intriguing. Veterinary medicine sources don't provide comment on this, so I would guess the answer is no, not like humans. If you consider how animals behave, they often go hide and nest. Unlike humans, who run 24/7 to be productive, animals sort of veg out, so to speak. Female animals build the place or nest, where they will give birth. They stay close to home.

Research by the late Dr. Herbert L. Borrison at Dartmouth Medical School showed that not all animals vomit. This is fascinating work because tests for drugs used for nausea and vomiting control won't show the same effects on all creatures.

Besides humans, dogs respond to all known agents that cause vomiting, and cats respond to most. Both pigs and monkeys respond selectively. Sheep, horses, and rats don't vomit at all. Rabbits might look like they are going to vomit, but they don't. Frogs only vomit in the summer, and chickens get diarrhea.

What's even more interesting is what queasy animals eat to settle their stomachs. Given that rats—as we've just learned—don't vomit, a Japanese group of researchers put 72 rats in rotation devices and spun them around and eventually watched their behaviors. (One would probably agree that spinning would induce nausea). While these researchers were studying the effects of various agents on the rats, they used an amount of kaolin (which is clay) as a proxy for the presumed queasiness. They found that the amount of clay eaten differed as they varied the combination of antinausea agents. This was fascinating information for me, because in many less-developed countries, pregnant women eat clay in response to morning sickness.

SMELLS THAT CALM FEMALE ANIMALS

We don't really know how animals really react to smells. However, they obviously do react. Researchers from Auburn University in Alabama found that a few spritzes of anise (licorice-flavored) oil makes dairy cows calmer, and, as a result, they produce more milk. If a good smell does it for Bossy, you know there has to be something to calm humans!

Chapter 6

Dealing with the Triggers for Morning Sickness

PEGGY

When Peggy and her husband were considering a third child, she phoned me for a consultation to find out what was new in the way of morning-sickness management. Three years earlier I had met this attractive but ashen woman in the check-out line at the grocery store. It was an odd place to encounter a potential client, but long, slow lines create an opportunity to talk to your grocery-wagon comrades. Her cart was filled with disposable diapers along with a hefty variety of microwave meals: This spelled postpartum to me. She looked so ill that I wondered if she was going to collapse on the spot. I asked her if she was all right, and said if it would help, we could swap places. I asked her if she was a new mother. She said yes, but it had been a horrible pregnancy with "wall to wall hyperemesis."

Walking out to our respective parked cars, she saw the panels on the side of my car—www.morningsickness.net—and promptly called me the "mobile morning-sickness maven"!

Because I hadn't taken care of her in either of her previous two pregnancies, Madison or Charlie, it would be important to dig through events that occurred in both. We'd need to review all events in each pregnancy to try to come up with a game plan for Baby #3. How similar had her other pregnancies been? What were the differences? Time of year? Living location?

When we tried to sort out the triggers that might affect Peggy in another pregnancy, heightened senses emerged as a major theme. Environmental issues were a problem, because she seemed to have acquired chemical sensitivities syndrome also. Peggy didn't remember as many details from her first pregnancy as from her second. She had had more opportunity to sleep through the first one without the added stress of taking care of a household. She said her memory of events during the first pregnancy was a "big blur." Maybe she wanted to deliberately forget about it all! She wasn't sure.

In both pregnancies Peggy recalled feelings of being "suffocated" by a hot shower if she used a perfumed soap. She was trying to figure out what cleaning agents she could use without going into a fit of coughing, which would then result in vomiting. This, being a problem when she was not pregnant, would undoubtably get worse with pregnancy.

Sexual intimacy could become a major problem—or rather the lack of it. Peggy's husband, Vinny, was not accustomed to being celibate. Although he could appreciate issues of vomiting, he had a hard time accepting "no, not now, I'm nauseous" over and over again. During one tense night of rebuffs, Vinny shouted, "this is about as much fun as a root canal!" and left to sleep in the guest room. Peggy felt guilty, but was actually relieved that the tension, for the moment, had been reduced. Previous to this nausea business, they enjoyed a healthy sex life. The thought of contact now—yikes—was enough to make her vomit! (And it had last weekend!) Just the wiggling around on the bed was enough to send Peggy over the edge.

Peggy recently learned that she was sensitive to wheat and gluten (see the appendix for a list of some wheat-free and gluten-free products). This food allergy might have been present to some degree with her second pregnancy, during which she had had a more than frantic quest to buy the "magic, right crackers." She had vomited up all the crackers she'd ever bought. Rice cakes seemed to work better than any cracker. Her nose was so sensitive she could smell the cardboard boxes when she opened the kitchen cupboards at home.

Doing the household laundry was a problem. This seemed to be a bigger problem with the second pregnancy. The old washer made a whiney, high-pitched noise during the spin cycle. Running the vacuum to pick up after a 2-year-old toddler, Madison, and her trail of Cheerios made her dizzy and exhausted. Vinny liked a clean and tidy house. But week after week, she lost ground with keeping up with a 2-year-old and a 10-room house and yard work. She eventually collapsed, seriously dehydrated from trying to mow the lawn.

She was hospitalized, in a small community facility with very few private rooms. After a three day stay in a room with three people, she begged her husband to get her a private room. It was only a 1-night stay, but finally she was able to sleep!

Peggy told me that she had been visited during her second pregnancy by the hospital psychiatrist while she was in the triple room, and she found that most distressing. She knew he was investigating her commitment to her pregnancy. Each time he said, "Well, she says she wants another baby . . . but I wonder what else is going on at home."

In trying to pinpoint factors contributing to the waxing and waning course of her morning sickness in the hospital, Peggy commented that every time she looked better, someone seemed to expect her to run laps around the floor. She found herself losing ground when she walked laps just before her wing of the hospital received meal trays, or when the housekeepers' dirty water buckets came too close.

One weekend, a part-time nurse told Peggy to empty her own emesis (vomit) basin after measuring and recording the contents on the I/O (intake/output) sheet. Shortly thereafter, she overheard a conversation between this older nurse and a student nurse. "I just hate emptying emesis basins," the older nurse said. "It always makes me sick, and I start to gag. I make them do it. After all, they have to do it at home. They should be used to it by now!"

Peggy was also asked to measure her urine and record the amount. She found the smell of her concentrated urine obnoxious. But she did not have the courage or stamina to tell the nurse that these tasks bordered on torture.

Peggy eventually recovered from her morning sickness and had a healthy second baby, Charlie. Peggy had tried to keep a journal during her second pregnancy, after watching other women journal over the course of their pregnancies. We reviewed her entries page by page, looking at all the events she jotted down and brainstorming about what might be done differently. We made long lists, referencing previous situations. It seemed to be a helpful encounter. In the end, Peggy decided she just couldn't do it again. She'd forgotten a lot of the bad times of being in bed, looking like death warmed over. She and Vinny enjoyed their wonderful children and family events. Vinny came from a large family, and all of his siblings had four to five kids; Vinny wanted more. Everything had been reviewed: medications, health care staff, hydration, and home and child-care issues. In the end, they thought about the required emotional stamina on both sides. Reluctantly, Vinny agreed: He didn't have the energy to take care of two kids and a sick wife for weeks on end, even though his family offered 24/7 help. In the end, Peggy and Vinny decided not to conceive a third child.

By now, you probably have a fairly good perspective on the variable nature of morning sickness. Nevertheless, if you're suffering from nausea or vomiting, getting through today requires significant emotional fortitude. If your case is severe, the promise of improved overall stability is a critical aspect. But that promise may seem out of reach.

Many women reluctantly admit that it's difficult to think about continuing a pregnancy when doing so means disability, misery, and suffering alone. Society's attitude—reflected in remarks like "oh, it's nothing to worry about" and "be glad you're pregnant"—has a lot to do with a woman's ability to cope.

As discussed in the previous chapter, even hospital care doesn't necessarily bring a cure and can carry its own special disruptions and ignominies. This chapter is a package of hints and encouragements to help you get through your morning sickness.

STIMULI: GOOD, BAD OR IN-BETWEEN

Are there smells that seem more acute during your pregnancy than before it and that add to your nausea? Are the smells temporary or permanent? Do you feel queasy because you've just awakened? Was the wake-up slow and gentle or startling? Are the lights too bright? Is there noise? If so, is it loud and irksome? What noise in particular is most irritating. Can it be reduced? Does it originate in your household, or is it beyond your immediate control? If you're not vomiting and you look fairly well, are you expected to perform either housework or office work? Do you feel pressure? From whom? Is your gastric distress the result of taking a prenatal vitamin, iron supplement, or medication? Or is it because you didn't take an antinausea medication on schedule?

Noise and Saliva

The excessive saliva that accompanies some women's morning-sickness experience is both a curiosity to health professionals and a pain in the neck to the women who try to cope with it. Besides the various properties in saliva—minerals and growth factors—the production of saliva is an interesting phenomenon. The average healthy person produces about 3 pints of saliva a day.

Research in saliva is facinating, although not particularly common. Some psychology researchers studied a group of nonpregnant people and found that those who were introverts produced more saliva than the extroverts when lemon juice was applied to the tongues of people in both groups. The explanation for why was thought to be connected to the sense of arousal, but this was not determined conclusively.

Researchers in Glasgow, Scotland, designed an experiment on college students that tested the amount of saliva produced in a quiet setting and then in a very noisy environment. For baseline, they collected the amount of saliva on a cotton swab that was placed over one of the salivary glands. Then another swab was placed in the same location and four drops of fresh lemon juice was applied to their tongues. Each of the 24 students was tested four times.

This experiment was then repeated in the presence of a noise that was considered "just too loud for comfort." This level of noise was selected individually by each study subject. What researchers found was that there was an increase in saliva production with increased levels of noise.

Granted, researchers have not conducted this experiment on any pregnant women, but the results of these studies may be applicable to pregnant women with morning sickness. If you are generally a quiet type, you may respond to stressful situations with an increase in saliva production. However, the connection to a noisy environment bears some attention. Noisy environments often increase stress levels, and stress levels are often accompanied by increases in bad stress hormone levels—notably cortisol. No one needs a lot of chronic cortisol floating around in their body, let alone a pregnant woman! The bottom line is, when your morning sickness is starting, even small amounts of noise may increase your level of discomfort—so find a quiet environment and go rest!

A few years ago, the *Wall Street Journal* ran an article about a device the U.S. military had used for crowd control in Bosnia. When directed at the rioters, the device caused them to be nauseated. So, clearly, certain frequencies or noise levels can cause nausea.

BAD WEATHER

Although there has been no formal investigation about the connection between bad weather and morning sickness that I know of, I've often been told by women that they are affected by weather changes. One plausible explanation is that lowered barometric pressure traps bad air, so there are more pollutants around to avoid. Making an expectant mother queasy during bad weather may be a way that Mother Nature forces a mother to seek cleaner environs to protect her unborn child. People with migraines seem to react adversely prior to an onslaught of bad weather as well. There is some suggestion that the stress hormone cortisol might be increased during these times of inclement weather. A researcher at the University of Connecticut, Lawrence E. Armstrong, reports there is evidence that a fluctuating balance of positive and negative ions in the air, especially in the wind, is to blame. Armstrong says the positive ions are the bad guys and can affect brain chemistry by altering the secretion of cortisol. You cannot change the weather, but it is helpful to know that there might be some connection so that you can keep an eye on weather patterns and then reduce your activity level to try to compensate.

Several years ago at my hospital, we started to look at weather patterns and the downhill slide some of our patients with morning sickness were experiencing. I was taking care of two severely sick women who had suffered large weight losses and were on intravenous nutrition at discharge from the hospital. Both were given weather homework to see if there was any correlation between their sickness and the weather. They were to report back to us periodically after a crash in their health. When they brought back their observations, we then looked at all the events that preceded the crash. The pattern that seemed to emerge fairly consistently was a negative change in the weather about 1.5 to 2 days before their downward spiral. One woman lived in the Worcester area and one on the South Shore in Boston. What we seemed to observe was that when Mrs. Worcester has heading for a decline, the weather in eastern Ohio and western Pennsylvania was horrible. Mrs. South Shore—pregnant with twin girls—would start to crumble when the weather in the Virginia–New Jersey area was nasty. These observations suggest these women somehow could sense bad weather coming along about 24 to 36 hours before it arrived on their door steps. This phenomenon is similar to canaries in the mines. Both of these weather women had female fetuses, which adds another interesting dimension to their morning sickness.

In case you aren't acquainted with the use of canaries in mines, I'll relate here an interesting story told to me by a mining engineer from South Africa. In the days before the advent of oxygen sensors, miners would take caged canaries into mines. More sensitive to oxygen depletion than humans, the canaries would start to act bizarre long in advance of oxygen depletion. Their behavior sounded the alarm and saved the miners from succumbing to carbon monoxide poisoning.

INDOOR POLLUTANTS

As the environmental temperature goes up, it's easier to become dehydrated, so keeping up with fluid requirements is more important than ever. When the bad weather is associated with a cold front, consider how people generally handle the situation: They close windows and turn up the heat. As a result, household smells can become more concentrated. Although you cannot see internal pollutants as easily, they do exist. Carpets, cabinets, paints, and many other household items emit volatile organic compounds (VOC). Included in this list of VOC-emitting items are fabric protection agents, which can contribute chemicals to your environment. One of my favorite publications, *Natural Home* does a super job of providing information about various household dangers and solutions (check out their Web site at www.naturalhomemagazine.com). Phylates and other agents in perfumes and fragrances are also bad for your health; however, you won't easily find information about these ingredients on labels. For more information on indoor polution, contact the Environmental Working Group in Washington, D.C., a consumer watch-dog organization. Write to them at Environmental Working Group 1436 U Street, NW Washington, D.C. 20009 or check them out online at www.ewg.org

One final interesting note on this topic, medical literature indicates that there seems to be a higher incidence of hospital admission in the Southeast, where the climate is often more hot and humid.

EATING AND SLEEPING

When you go to bed, try to keep a window open at least 1 to 2 inches—unless, of course, noise is a problem or security is an issue. You might consider getting a small fan to provide soothing white noise. A well-ventilated room should decrease stale bedroom air in the morning. (One of the hospitalized women I cared for found the odor from a new vinyl mattress so offensive that she had her husband bring in swimmer's nose clips.) If you've been vomiting in the middle of the night, wait at least 1 or 2 hours after your last meal before going to sleep. Otherwise, eating until you fall asleep will presumably reduce the likelihood of low blood sugar on waking, which some sources claim causes nausea. Again, the watchword is do what feels best.

If you're exhausted and want to sleep immediately after eating, try lying on your right side. This may help empty your stomach faster, because the stomach empties from left to right. If you lie on your left side, your stomach must pump food uphill. Lying on the left side also seems to pool the stomach contents directly below the end of the esophagus. Because the tone of the esophageal sphincter muscle is thought to be relaxed by the presence of pregnancy hormones, it may be less effective in keeping the contents of the stomach contained.

Some books tell you not to eat right before going to bed, because it may disturb your sleep. Eating or drinking some foods or beverages does cause a problem for some women. The most common culprit is caffeine, found in coffee, tea, colas, and chocolate. But another substance, phenylethylamine, is also found in these items, as well as in aged cheeses, sausages, and pickled herring. Phenylethylamine can constrict small blood vessels, which can aggravate headaches and disturb rest.

Monosodium glutamate (MSG) is also reported to increase brain activity and heart rate in some people, which can disturb sleep. Commonly found in Chinese restaurant food, MSG also turns up in Mexican, French, American, and Italian dishes, as well as in many prepared grocery store foods. The tastier the food, the likelier it contains MSG. Sauerkraut, meat tenderizers, and bouillon cubes contain lots of MSG. Sometimes it's disguised on the label as "natural flavorings" or hydrolyzed vegetable protein (HVP). My own experience is that MSG in a spicy evening meal will cost me more hours of sleep than several cups of coffee.

If you have success with certain foods, and the nutrients they contain (rather than their tastes or textures) seem to be the connecting factor, stay with that approach. If you need more individual nutrient analysis, contact a registered dietitian (R.D.) who has a computerized nutrient-analysis program. For those of you who have food allergies, look for cookbooks that will allow others to make whatever food you need without the offending ingredient. One such book is The Complete Allergy Cookbook written by Marylin Gioannini.

CAUTION SIGNS

It's often easier to relay information about a possible change in your condition to others in advance than at the beginning of a crisis. To that end, I've created a few signs for you to post near your hospital bed, at home, in the office, or wherever you're staying.

Most women I've worked with have said that when they feel the worst it's easiest just to say, "I'm doing what the doctor/dietitian books say to do." The following signs can be copied and enlarged on a copy machine or clipped out of the book. In fact, you might want to have a copy of the book where family, friends, or coworkers can pick it up and learn more about what you're going through.

Danger/Danger/Danger

Danger/Danger

Sensitive Nose Ahead!

Unstable Stomach Condition

VOMITING COULD OCCUR

Smell Watch/ Smell Watch/ Smell Watch

FOR THE OFFICE

WARNING/WARNING/WARNING

WARNING/WARNING

Right now my sense of smell is extremely sensitive, so I'd appreciate it if you *WOULDN'T*

1. Sit too close to me.
2. Bring your coffee cup within 20 feet of my desk.
3. Breathe on me.
4. Wear too much cologne, perfume, or aftershave.
5. Use any cleaning agents or sprays or bring wash pails close to my area.
6. Leave the coffeepot on all day.
7. Smoke close to me.
8. _____
9. _____

Both my baby and I thank you for your compassion and sensitivity.

FOR THE HOUSEHOLD AND ANY GUESTS

> ### WARNING: FRAGILE HOSTESS AHEAD
>
> 1. Welcome to this humble home.
> 2. Please acquaint yourself with the kitchen, dishes, stove, refrigerator, and sink.
> 3. Presently I am suffering from an ancient ailment: motherhood miseries, a.k.a. morning sickness (in extreme cases, hyperemesis gravidarum).
> 4. Primary symptom: Radar nose. I smell everything.
> 5. Please wash your own dishes, clean up after yourself, and do not use perfume, cologne, aftershave, or hairspray in, this house.
> 6. Please don't smoke in my house or in my car.
> 7. To get brownie points, you can offer to change my other child's diapers, take the trash out, feed the cat, or change the litter box (circle what applies).
>
> (Fill in further requests) _____
>
> Both my baby and I appreciate your understanding and help in reducing the factors that add to the uncontrollable problems of nausea (and vomiting).

TRACKING THE GOOD AND BAD TIMES

Another question to ask and answer is what time of day is most associated with nausea or vomiting? Is the time of day the only factor, or is there a contributing factor (physical or emotional) from something or someone else? Rating the degree of nausea from 1 to

10 (1 being the worst) at various times, along with foods or beverages requested, has been helpful for several women. Recording these data on the chart in Figure 6.1 may present you with a clearer picture of how to approach each day. Before recording any information on the chart, make several copies of the blank sheets for future use.

Figure 6.1

Time	Score 1–10	Level of Smells	Amount of Motion	Level of Noise	Preference/ Taste	Texture of Food Eaten	Quality of Climate

The tracking sheet is basically a journal of your progress. There are several variables that most women consider negative, all involving the senses (smell, motion, noise, and climate); these appear at the top of the page.

The times at which you take medication, eat, or drink can make a big difference. The duration of any average activity can be a make-or-break factor. Once you're aware that everything affects your gastric stability and you plot all the variables, a pattern generally emerges. A rating scale of 1 (worst) to 10 (best) can help pinpoint positive and negative factors.

Record any and all variables, because that's the only way to analyze both the invisible trigger and stabilizer factors. Various foods and beverages will probably have a predictable pattern of appeal once you've compiled the rest of the data.

You may note that the presence or absence of humidity in the morning can set the tone for the day. One woman discovered that when humidity was high in the morning her day's activity was minimal. However, when the morning was much less humid, her activity increased dramatically by early afternoon. She also learned that overactivity in the afternoon resulted in a crash by early evening, a crash that lasted for the next 2 or 2 1/2 days. Once this trend was spotted and discussed, she tapered her activities on low-humidity days and prevented the recurrence of crashes.

Keeping a food diary can be extremely helpful, too. Recipes considered as well as those used or modified should be noted. This may help you or others zero in on future food possibilities.

TRACKING SHEET EXAMPLE: SUSIE AND FRED

During Susie's pregnancy, she kept a tracking sheet to identify her triggers for morning sickness. Comparing Susie's narrative with her tracking sheet, in Figure 6.2, shows how she tracked events throughout the day. For example, Susie's tracking sheet notes that her husband Fred's tossing and turning resulted in his facing and breathing on her as soon as she woke up. This set off her morning sickness, which she rated 1, or really bad. She found that after vomiting she regained some of her composure by sitting in the cool morning air on the back porch; she rated this 3. She wanted something cold, textured, and bland to settle her stomach and found relief with a rice cake and a small amount of ice chips (made from distilled water and stored in the freezer in a sealed plastic bag). She felt a bit weak and continued to rate her condition 3.

Susie was just beginning to feel as if she could dress when Fred decided to turn on the news. The sudden loud sound made her jump and become tense, maintaining her 3 status. Susie yelled at Fred to turn down the volume and decided to keep sitting on the porch for another 20 minutes. She blew Fred a kiss through the screen door and asked him not to hug her, because he'd put on aftershave. She ate a few more ice chips and decided to go inside and dress. Fred had

---

Figure 6.2

6 a.m. 1: Wake up Fred breathed on me.

7 a.m. 3: Sat on porch—clean air. Bland rice cake (want dry textured food).

8 a.m. 3: No noise! Fred turned on the news loudly!

9 a.m. 4: Dog food! (in kitchen) to porch again.

10 a.m. 5: Feel better. Tent dress. Drove to work.

11 a.m. 6: Sat in office—Door closed. Ate ham and cheese sandwich.

Noon. 3!: Old coffee pot & muggy stale air in boss's office.

1 p.m. 5: Ate fresh orange & raw carrots (want crunch & sweet).

2 p.m. 7: Craving ice cream—frozen yogurt OK but not quite "it" (want cold & sweet).

3 p.m. 7–*6: Getting tired—better leave early!

4 p.m. 5: Pooped. Opened refrigerator at home! Smell of old food.

5 p.m. 8: Feel better. Called Fred to get "to go" food and eat outside on porch.

---

put canned food out for the dog, Mugzie, and after one step into the house, Susie retreated to the porch for more fresh air and hopes of maintaining a slightly improved rating of 4. She ate a few more ice chips.

An hour later, at a score of 5, Susie had a shower, dressed uneventfully, and drove to work with a prepacked lunch bag that contained an air-sickness bag, a clean, wet facecloth, and fresh lemon. The stop-and-go motion in the parking garage and the closed-up feeling caused low-level queasiness, which Susie was able to ward off by smelling the lemon. When she parked her car, she took a drink of the cold seltzer she carried in her cooler. She noted her gastrointestinal status as 6.

Susie arrived at her desk after the coffee break and before lunch so that food smells were at a low level. She promptly ate a ham and cheese sandwich, and at lunchtime headed out for a walk to avoid cafeteria food smells. She'd made progress: She now rated her condition at 6. Because the sun was bright, she wore sunglasses and walked with her friend Millie, who respected her need for peace and quiet. The ham and cheese sandwich and the walk made Susie thirsty, so she made herself a "brown cow" (half cola and half low-fat milk) at the snack bar in the cafeteria. She was free of nausea, a 6, until she was on her way back to her office desk, when she felt instantly queasy. Looking around, she spied a filmy coffeepot with 1 inch of well-cooked coffee. Her status plummeted to 3. She ran to the bathroom, losing part of her lunch. She then sat with a cold facecloth on her forehead while crunching on ice chips.

About an hour later Susie had recovered to about a 5 and wanted something crunchy and sweet, which she decided would be a fresh orange and carrot sticks. Her old officemate Liz stopped by for a chat, but Liz's newest perfume made Susie bolt out of her chair and down the hall for fresh air. When she felt better, she said as diplomatically as possible, "Liz, no offense to you but your perfume and my stomach just aren't going to be buddies." Two cups of ice-cold water with a twist of lime, sipped slowly, went down well, boosting her fluid total for the day so far to 5 1/4 cups, or slightly over half of the "stay-even" allowance set by her prenatal nutritionist.

At 2 p.m. Susie's taste buds asked for vanilla ice cream, with a rating of 7. She was marginally satisfied after having to settle for vanilla frozen yogurt. The office had warmed up now that the sun was pouring through the window, and Susie felt the need to shed her shoes and plant her feet on the bare wooden floor. The sweetness of the yogurt made her thirsty, and she decided a cold can of ginger ale from the vending machine might be called for. Twelve ounces later she continued to feel well, or at 7.

By 3 p.m. Susie felt a decline setting in and decided to leave early to avoid a crash in the office. She drove with the car windows open until she was passed by a Greyhound bus, when she hurriedly closed the windows. Twenty minutes later she turned into the driveway of her new ranch house. Opening the refrigerator door proved to be a mistake; the smell of Fred's leftover takeout dinner leaped out and instantly provoked nausea and a dry retch or two. An hour's nap saved the afternoon. By 5 p.m. Susie had called Fred's office, suggesting he bring home another takeout dinner for two, and they would dine on the back porch while the sun set. Fred arrived home with dinner for two, picked up at the local deli, and found Susie munching on a grilled cheese and tomato sandwich Mrs. Jones from next door had delivered. Susie hadn't been able to wait. Fred smiled and shrugged.

As you can see from Susie's chart, there were numerous variables that needed to be identified quickly. Both negative and positive factors differed in their impact. Only by regularly listing key events will you be able to take defensive action. Listen to the messages you're hearing from your body.

Chapter 7

A Candid Look at Feelings: Emotions and Morning Sickness

ALAN AND CLAIRE

When Alan and Claire received the official news that she was pregnant, they had already endured a week of sporadic nausea and vomiting. Soon after, Claire spent a weekend in the hospital. Alan's method of coping was to begin smoking again, after a 6-year hiatus. He found talking to people unhelpful and believed that very few understood what he was experiencing. Almost everyone seemed to say "it's just normal morning sickness." He spent all his free time visiting Claire in the hospital. Too worried to relax, he avoided direct questions from family and friends and would often change the subject. He was a licensed psychologist, so he was supposed to know more about coping than the average person, or so he'd always been told. But being part of it up close and personal was an experience he had not trained for during his PhD work. Alan finally decided that he was in a position to learn something new during this time of adversity and started to keep notes about the events, his feelings, and his reactions. He contributed to the dad's forum on the www.helpher.org Web site.

He was particularly irritated one day when he made lunch for Claire, something he executed with culinary finesse—a grilled cheese and tomato sandwich. It was a perfect sandwich. However, he'd been weeding and planting in the garden earlier and had dirt under his fingernails. All Claire could focus on was the dark line of earth on and under his fingernails. She was instantly repulsed and felt a huge wave of nausea overtake her. She put her hands over her face and said weakly, "I just can't eat that now." It had taken her days to tell Alan that he smelled really awful when he took his fish-oil capsules. That piece of news hadn't gone down easily. Now, the dirty fingernails—how and when was she going to deliver that headline event? She knew she had to, because she couldn't afford to not to eat and keep throwing up over triggers she knew were lethal to her stomach. She figured if she found an article in the newspaper about soil-borne bacteria in the *New York Times* or *Wall Street Journal,* her job would be made easier.

Claire found the information she was looking for, after logging onto the Internet. Soil contains all sorts of nasty parasites that can cause disease and fetal damage. The list is long but real. Because of the potential of fetal damage, women are advised to wash raw vegetables well before eating. Even fruits, such as cantaloupe and watermelon, which might not look dirty, can contain *E. coli* bacteria, which can be imparted to the surface of fruit by a knife that becomes contaminated from the outside surface. Parsley, alfalfa sprouts, and other salad greens that can be hard to wash have been known to carry bad bugs.

The article also commented on checking out the bathrooms of restaurants before you order your meal. If it's dirty, stop and think about the hygiene in the kitchen. And if the wait staff has dirty nails or hands, you might talk to the manager and take your appetite elsewhere. Claire also read about leaving your gardening shoes outside in the garage to reduce the amount of potential contamination in your house. This is especially important when your baby turns toddler—becomes a rug rat—and crawls all over your house. Even if you don't have a garden, leaving your shoes at the door, as is the custom in Japan, makes a lot of sense. Street dirt can also contain fragments of lead dust, from leaded gas. Besides that, why track in more dirt and grime that you'll have to vacuum up later anyway? Slippers by the door are the answer, and your house will be quieter as a result.

Alan liked the idea about house slippers. He even found a few bargain pairs for guests to wear. As a side benefit, he noticed fewer scratch marks on their expensive, antique dining room furniture. After his experience, Alan had some advice for other men: "Talk to your wife about your feelings, her fears, both of your thoughts about the baby, and about pregnancy in general. After all, this is a major life event! There will be time in the future for happiness and fun, but do not expect anything for a while until your wife is feeling better." (By "expect anything," Alan meant sexual intimacy.)

THE EMOTIONS OF PREGNANCY

If you're a miserable mother-to-be, the waxing and waning emotions you might experience can range through the following (and beyond):

Anger—You may be angry that you're so sick and that others may expect standard, everyday well-person performance. Or you may be angry with yourself because of disappointed expectations. Your anger may be directed at your doctor and your insurance company for not making it easier to get care. You may even be angry at your mate for getting you pregnant with problems!

Guilt—You may feel guilty because you resent the disruption of your life by morning sickness. Your guilt may be because the pregnancy was unplanned and you must decide whether to continue it. You may have guilt about wanting to eat but being unable to.

Uncertainty—Maybe you feel uncertain about how long your job, other commitments, and your whole life will stay on hold because of morning sickness, which makes getting through a day a full-time job in itself. You may have uncertainty about continuing the pregnancy because everyone is asking, "How come you're so sick?" or because of financial worries.

Isolation—You may feel isolated because none of the several dozen books about pregnancy you've flipped through discussed morning sickness in detail. You may begin to think, "I must be the only person who ever feels like this! What's wrong with me?" Everyone you meet seems to say in total amazement, "Gee, I never met anyone before who has what you have!"

Exhaustion—You never feel or look rested even though you seem to sleep all the time. The bags under your eyes are sagging toward your knees. Your disposition may deteriorate. Plans to go anywhere with anyone are on permanent hold because you never know whether it'll be a good day or a bad day. By now friends may not be calling so often.

Fear—You may be afraid the nausea and vomiting will never end. Particularly, if you've never been this sick before, it can be tough to believe that this isn't something more than morning sickness. You may not be convinced your doctor is totally competent—if he or she was, wouldn't you be better by now? Perhaps you are afraid you will die or have some permanent problem as a result of morning sickness or hyperemesis.

Recurrent thoughts of food—People who are starving often have thoughts of food and eating. This is not uncommon, but why it happens can only be speculated. Food is a pleasure—starving is painful. Perhaps the brain is trying to compensate in some way.

Forgetfulness—Forgetfulness comes with starvation and lack of important nutrients and calories to keep the brain going.

Abandonment—Who stays around when your nausea and vomiting are at their worst? Perhaps the only person who'll really understand is your mother, maybe because mothers have gone through a lot of mess and unpleasantness in their time. But if there are bumps in your relationship with your mother, smoothing them out in the middle of your physical crisis may be a tough job.

Betrayal—Maybe your spouse or significant other says, "It's all in your head," or, "This could stop if you really tried," then announces that he can't be much help anyway and goes about his usual activities. Because your situation is partly his doing, you may be upset that he isn't around when you need him.

Unattractiveness—The best you can seem to do now is open you eyes in the morning. Makeup may be totally out of the picture. You've heard you're supposed to glow, but it's tough to be radiant in baggy sweats with filmy teeth and oily skin. Nobody ever mentioned that this might be part of the deal.

Vulnerability—Although you are likely to feel vulnerable during your pregnancy, your spouse may be feeling vulnerable, too. Some men who have seen family members, especially their mothers, become terminally ill find it difficult to cope with a woman suffering from nausea and vomiting. Seeing you bedridden can generate an overwhelming foreboding and sense of vulnerability, which saps energy and is difficult to surmount alone.

PREGNANCY AND THE COMPLICATIONS OF EATING DISORDERS

The amount of body fat a woman has may affect her hormone levels and, hence, her ability to get pregnant. Women who are underweight as well as those who are overweight are at risk for infertility. For the overweight woman, losing a few pounds might mean getting pregnant without intervention. Weight loss in an overweight woman is usually a positive situation, although it may be difficult for some women who struggle with eating disorders such as binge eating. For an underweight woman, being asked to gain 10 pounds is a difficult proposition. This is especially true for those with eating disorders such as anorexia or bulimia. In Western culture, the prevailing attitude is "thin is in and stout is out." So some thin, underweight, or athletic women who have a difficult time getting pregnant naturally because of a low percentage of body fat, resist weight gain and often opt for invasive reproductive help.

Some women who have had eating disorders get pregnant naturally, but many only become pregnant with the help of modern advanced reproduction technology. Many of them suffer from morning sickness as well. In addition to the physical discomforts, women who have had eating disorders may experience additional stress when dealing with morning sickness. Vomiting from morning sickness may not be easily distinguished from the vomiting that accompanies the binge-purge syndrome known as bulimia. In fact, a case of self-induced vomiting by an ex-bulimic woman, who was also pregnant, has been noted in the medical literature under a syndrome called bulimia nervosa. Unfortunately, it is unclear whether the woman was also suffering from morning sickness and could have been merely trying to find relief. One researcher also found that 17 percent of women who attended infertility clinics had histories of eating disorders that were undetected. Eating disorders are very complicated and can include complex family dynamics. The topic is beyond the scope of this book, but anyone with a history of eating disorders needs to get help before becoming pregnant. Women with histories of eating disorders compounded by bad morning sickness are at risk for poorer pregnancy outcomes. Cesarean deliveries and lower birth weights are more common because of poor nutritional status. The increased rate of cesarean deliveries is *not* due to large-sized babies but rather is due to babies who might have poor fetal testing during pregnancy. If a doctor thinks the baby is not thriving or moving adequately—for whatever reason—sometimes emergency deliveries are ordered to ensure a live baby.

Talk to your doctor about it if you have a history of eating disorders. Depression is often a component of eating disorders. Changing your diet might also help with the depression. Omega-3 fatty acids have been found in certain studies to be helpful in combating depression. Omega-3 fatty acids are found in fatty fishes, flaxseeds, flaxseed oil, walnuts, and farm-raised wild game fed diets high in omega-3 fatty acids. A good book on the topic is *The Omega 3 Connection*, by Dr. Andrew Stoll.

Separating symptoms of morning sickness from symptoms of eating disorders seems to be especially difficult for women who have cured themselves of their eating disorders through self-help, because they may lack the reinforcement of others who might note a change in behavior and attitude. A woman's knowledge that her body is about to change radically is often a major concern, and some professionals feel that certain women have great difficulty accepting this fact, especially the super-fit and athletically minded.

Some women with no prior history of purge-type eating disorders have resorted to self-induced vomiting to ease morning sickness. One pregnant woman at my hospital who reported episodes of self-induced vomiting was suspected of having an underlying eating disorder. However, when I met with her, I found a thoroughly exhausted woman merely trying to find relief from the never-ending nausea. She said that she was unable to leave her home for fear that eventually she would vomit in front of others. Although few women admit this concern, it is seems understandable, especially because women report that once they vomit, the sensations of nausea are gone . . . for a while.

In 1 week, 2 hospitalized women with severe morning sickness reluctantly admitted self-induced vomiting to me. They believed that few people would be sympathetic to their miseries, and both worried about being branded weird. One woman was being harassed by her husband's family because he had told them she made herself vomit. She was not only angry with him but desperate for relief, since she had had a previous abortion because of similar illness. One study found 60 percent of 43 women considering abortion had had nausea with retching or vomiting.

INTRAVENOUS FLUIDS AND PANIC ATTACKS

One woman told me that during her pregnancy she had to go to a busy emergency room by herself to receive intravenous fluids. She reported "freaking out." She wasn't sure what the fluid was or whether there was any medicaiton in it, but she thought she heard somone refer to it as *lactated ringers*. Her sensation of "freaking out" might have been a type of panic reaction. She reported no history of recognized panic disorder, but I'm not a psychiatrist and would not know what kind of exploratory questions to pose.

There are three basic types of fluids one can get when hydration is needed:

- D5, which is 5 percent dextrose (or sugar) in water.
- NS, which is normal saline (or 9 percent salt—sodium and chloride) in water.
- LR, or lactated ringers, which is salt—sodium, chloride, and bicarbonate (bicarb)—in water. The bicarbonate part of this solution is helpful when one is acidotic, which is often the case when one is starving and spilling ketones. You use a form of bicarbonate when you cook—baking soda.

One can also get hybrids of the above three solutions. D5LR is a combination of sugar, salt, and bicarbonate. You can also get 1/2 NS, which is 4.5 percent salt.

Medical literature has mixed opinions on the role of lactated ringers solution and panic and anxiety problems, but it has been investigated. To date, there were no reports of lactated ringers solution, pregnancy, malnutrition, and panic issues. That doesn't mean some relationship doesn't exist. Whether panic attacks occur with other fluids has not been reported. The temperature of fluids might also be a factor in how people feel in the early minutes of hydration. If the fluid has just been taken out of the refrigerator, it will be going into the person's veins at about 35°F. I've heard women report shivering and having uncomfortable sensations with cold intravenous fluid administration. Once fluids reach room temperature, the level of discomfort may be minimized.

Certainly, in this woman's case, she experienced weight loss and malnutrition, so those variables are important to keep in mind. She was also alone in a very busy place. Being able to self-advocate when you are sick is a hard thing to do if you really have to investigate what is going on with your care. If she had taken a notebook with her and jotted down the events and processes that were going on, it would have been helpful in sorting out any connections.

One animal study showed that female sex hormones, estrogen in particular, increase vascular sensitivity to catecholamines, which are stress hormones. So, it is hard to say whether the lactated ringers solution produced the freaky feelings or whether it was a reaction to increased stress from all the action in the emergency department.

UNKNOWN ROOTS CAN BE PAINFUL

Pregnancy is a time of immense challenge and change, and all women long for the advise and comfort of their mothers. Adopted children not only have missed an important and vital part of their lives when they have been unable to meet their biological parents, but they also may not have access to their family's medical history. Some sick women have mothers who have had really bad morning sickness, and some have not. The anxiety morning sickness generates is bad enough—wondering about a missing parent doesn't help. This may be a time to seek spiritual guidance if it has not been sought before.

GETTING HELP

If you're having morning sickness and you feel isolated, seek out a sympathetic counselor to help you maintain your emotional equilibrium. Finding someone who has also experienced morning sickness and is sympathetic may be a Herculean task. A therapist with a waiting room full of clients may respond with revulsion if one of his or her patients suddenly retches or vomits.

A well-qualified counselor should be sympathetic to any situation, even if she or he has never shared the experience. The woman in need of additional emotional support has the option of shopping around if the initial contact proves unsatisfactory. No one should settle for the therapist recommended by the doctor's office if the match is wrong.

STAYING IN TOUCH

Becoming housebound because of the unpredictable nature of the morning-sickness problem is not unusual. Should this happen to you, telephone contact is vital. Because nausea and vomiting don't keep scheduled appointments of any sort, even telephone contact can become sporadic. To solve that problem, you should make it known beforehand that you may need to hang up abruptly. Some women find that talking is a way to keep nausea down; others find it to have just the opposite effect. One woman, whose job required a lot of personnel training and speaking before groups, said that after she'd talked for a long while it felt as though someone was pressing a finger into the back of her throat, and she suffered retching. We figured out that what was probably happening: Her gag reflex was probably more sensitive because of the prolonged tongue motion that occurs with talking. Certain places on the tongue are connected by the vagus (or wandering) nerve to various parts of body, notably the stomach. With increased pressure on these points, nausea can increase.

Every woman has her good window, or the time of the day when she feels somewhat improved. Sometimes talking just a few seconds after this improved time has passed is enough to escalate nausea and generate more saliva. Saliva, as you read about in Chapter 4, can trigger nausea. Sometimes merely talking about food becomes another trigger. Once you understand what may trigger nausea or vomiting, it's helpful to share your discoveries with others.

DOMESTIC VIOLENCE AND SHELTERS FOR SAFETY

The sick and sad truth is that domestic violence affects one in three women, according to data from the National Coalition against Domestic Violence. Four to eight percent of pregnant women experience violence during their pregnancies, making it more common than gestational diabetes, or preeclampsia, conditions routinely screened for in pregnant women by physicians. If a member of the household has anger-management problems, pregnancy may precipitate aggressive behavior toward the baby as relationships and roles change with the addition of a new member to the family.

Being sick makes one dependent upon others for care and, on occasion, one's partner may expose an ugly side of his personality when having to take on the role of nurturer and maid. Health-care providers are all required to screen for domestic violence, but it is a hard thing for a woman to admit. Being pregnant does not make admitting a violent relationship any easier because the woman may be worried about where she will go. Safe shelters do exist. Social workers in your health-care setting can help you, and your doctor wants to know about your safety concerns.

If you are having problems with domestic turmoil coupled with morning sickness, looking after yourself for the long haul might not be something you have energy to consider. Someone can help you. If you are in immediate danger, call 911. You can also call (800) 799-SAFE (7233) or log onto www.ncadv.org. If you do not have access to a computer at home, please go to your nearest library and ask the reference librarian to help you log on and learn how to find resources. Social workers in pregnancy clinics are also available to you, so please make contact if domestic violence is an issue for you. Your newborn is also at risk for abuse if you are.

HOMELESS SHELTERS

The reasons women live in homeless shelters are complex. The rules by which homeless shelters operate are also complicated and specific to each organization, according to one social worker I interviewed. I have cared for women from shelters who are hospitalized for hyperemesis. Their social supports are very limited, and their sense of hopelessness is great. Social workers are available to assist these women, but their resources are not endless. Like other women with bad morning sickness, the immediate environment plays a big role in keeping nausea and vomiting in check. These women improve dramatically with intravenous fluids, feeding individual foods on demand, and the peace and quiet of a private hospital room. However, there is no way to predict whether the cycle of nausea can be squelched successfully.

The resources available to other women with morning sickness to help in management are not easily accessed by homeless women. Many do not use libraries frequently, so they may have difficulty accessing books such as this one and Web sites for support. Your sensitivity to these women can help enormously. If you run into someone who is homeless or who works for a homeless shelter, you can do much to increase resource utilization by keeping in mind what you have just read. Your sensitivity could help change someone's life situation.

BOREDOM AND MORNING SICKNESS

Being homebound can generate both boredom and restlessness. The nausea decreases your attention span, yet distractions and activities remain necessary. Your chosen tasks should require a fair amount of concentration but probably not much thinking. Learning something new requires a degree of mental energy. If the activity is too grand in scope, it may generate mental stress and strain. Here are a few activities that do not require dollar investments or tremendous mental labors:

Making beaded barrettes or belts with a kit

Watching an ant farm and reading a children's book on what goes on in it

Watching birds at a feeder attached to the bedroom window

Writing a child's storybook for the baby's third or fourth birthday, complete with pictures

Stargazing with a telescope and star chart (if you don't get dizzy from this)

Turning doodles into greeting cards

Listening to books on tape (check your local library before going to the bookstore)

Reading short stories onto tapes to give to sight-impaired booklovers

Reading children's stories onto tapes for Christmas, birthday, or sick-day presents (these could be helpful for your baby-sitters in later years)

Planting flowers in a window box and watching them grow

Caring for goldfish or exotic fish

Origami—the Japanese art of paper folding

Watching educational videos

Rewriting your address book

Playing with Legos or Tinker Toys

Playing Scrabble or other word games

Making your own crossword puzzles for gifts

Organizing a photo album

Swapping activity lists with other women in your situation

Eating a fortune cookie a day and saving the fortunes

Clipping and saving your horoscope from the daily newspaper

Pressing any get-well flowers to frame later

Reading a great book, such as *A Natural History of the Senses,* by Diane Ackerman (if nothing else, the descriptions will generate laughter)

Listening to relaxation tapes

Listening to "Car Talk" (Click and Clack, the Tappet Brothers) on public radio (you don't have to have a car to enjoy this crazy show)

Making old-fashioned paper dolls and doll clothes for a local fund drive, such as the Salvation Army Christmas drive

Rereading the books you loved as a child

Knitting or embroidering

Starting a small herb garden using pots on a sunny windowsill (be sure to choose some that smell good to you)

There's a public charity on the Internet called HER Foundation. They provide emotional buddies. Contact them at info@hyperemesis.org. See www.helpher.org.

MORNING SICKNESS AND INTIMACY

It's important to address sexual issues in pregnancy; that is, sex is going to be on hold indefinitely. To date, there is only one article about sexuality in pregnancy that I could find, and it was a study from Nigeria. Five hundred women were studied. Sixty-four percent reported reduced sexual interest. Thirty percent avoided sexual intimacy because of the problem of nausea and vomiting, and 12 percent avoided it for fear of miscarriage.

Smells or odors of a bed partner, kissing, and motion—it's all there. Besides the chronic nausea issues, most women will have very tender breasts and complain that any pressure hurts. One of the theories about morning sickness, in fact, is that its evolutionary purpose is to discourage pregnant women from having sexual encounters! It has been speculated that the contractile force of an orgasm might disrupt the embryo's attachment to the uterine wall.

I have talked to enough green and queasy women to know that nausea and celibacy create escalating marital tension. You might want to talk with a social worker or your doctor if you feel your spouse is becoming emotionally abusive as the abstinence factor is prolonged.

I know of at least one situation in which a woman hospitalized for bad morning sickness decided to file for divorce and not return to her old house with her two kids. She was fed up with being sick but could do little about that. She was really fed up with the insensitivity of the father of her children, who expected her to take care of the house and the kids so he could go to work. As I recall, he worked two jobs and was totally worn out with the added burden of child care, grocery shopping, and housework. Whether they resolved their difficulties through marriage counseling I don't know. Perhaps earlier interventions, such as part-time nanny services, might have kept emotions from exploding. Nanny help can be expensive, but divorce and breaking up a household over morning sickness is tragic. Community services do exist. Contact your hospital department of social service or local church or synagogue and inquire about help if your supply of friends and family members has been exhausted.

MEDICAL BENEFIT OF SPIRITUALITY

Living in Boston, I've had the benefit of attending several places of worship for moving sermons and of enjoying the fabulous architecture inherent in these old buildings. One building that is particularly graceful in design is the Mother Church of the Christian Science Center on Mass Ave., a church founded by Mary Baker Eddy. After a tour of the building and library one day, I looked through her book *Guide to the Scriptures*, which covered many life aspects. She emphasized the importance of kindness, epsecially in health care, which is very important.

Dark Clouds, Silver Linings by Dr. Archibald D. Hart, published in 1993, is helpful in understanding how loss precipitates depression. And, certainly, women who are sick have losses—those of temporary health and of expectations of a fun pregnancy. Although this one book alone can't dig you out of a depression, it has steps about building self-esteem that are very positive and can be a place for you to start.

Prayer has been studied for its therapeutic potential by many outside of religious organizations. Dr. Larry Dossey is one such person. His book *Healing Words: The Power of Prayer and the Practice of Medicine* is a must-read. One chapter I found particularly inspiring was "Saints and Sinners, Health and Illness." He says if we look around in nature we would see that "plants, animals, birds, and fishes get sick, just as we do . . . yet when animals or plants get sick, we take a different attitude toward them. We do not judge or blame them. . . . [I]n nature the occurrence of disease is considered a part of the natural order, not a sign of ethnical, moral, or spiritual weakness."

When you are sick, reading can be difficult. Words of comfort are found in many corners, not just in church or a synagogue, but that's where we most expect to find them. One little pocket book I like is *The Reflecting Pond: Meditations for Self-Discovery*, by Liane Cordes. This book is published as part of the Hazelden Meditation Series.

A gem of a book to help make you cheerful is *2,002 Ways to Cheer Yourself Up*, by Cyndi Haynes. This book has something for everyone who needs an emotional hug. Here are two to consider: Number 140 "Whistle while you work. Hey it worked for the dwarfs!" and Number 1,017 "Keep in mind that everyone suffers from major life trials at one time or another. You are not unusual!"

I realize that thinking about the mode of deliver of this baby— vaginal versus cesarean delivery (equal surgery)—is probably light-years away from you. Nonetheless, your baby will be born one of two ways. One resource that is particularly helpful is Peggy Huddleston's book *Prepare for Surgery, Heal Faster*.

Men historically have been resistant to seeking help when stressed. They are as bewildered by all of this as you are. But they may not talk about it easily. Falling into old stress-reducing behaviors, such as smoking, is not uncommon. As sad as it is, some research suggests smoking has antidepressant properties.

GETTING NUTRITIONAL HELP

Certainly, being nutritionally compromised affects one's mental health and outlook. Depression is a common side effect of weight loss. There are a variety of nutrients needed daily, so finding something to eat is important: Comfort food or junk food works in some cases. See Chapter 12 for some nutrition ticklers.

TALK TO THE LEMONS!

As you read earlier, lemons can really help relieve depression. And using lemons for nausea does work. Sniff them, put them in water, lick them—whatever. Use lemontherapy all over the place. Cut up a fresh one every day and put it in a zippered plastic bag to smell at any time during the day. It can be a cheap way to get a quick fix of fresh air.

HELPFUL HUMOR

As I was researching updated material for this book, a new book came out on the topic of morning sickness: *The Morning Sickness Companion,* by Elizabeth Kaledin, who is a medical editor at CBS. One night I got on a crowded trolley in Brookline, heading home after a long day at work and pulled out this book to whip through a few more pages. Well, don't you know, some guy got up from his prime seat and said, "Hey, Ma'am, why don't you take my seat?" I thought, "geez, that's awfully nice of him! But I'm not hopping on crutches and don't think I look *that* exhausted tonight!" It then occurred to me he saw the cover of the book I was reading and probably thought I was about to heave all over 50 people squashed in that D-line train! I took the seat and figured that the book might be a real advantage in traveling and elsewhere! Ms. Kaledin offers another resource and levity to this miserable condition. I like the section on exercise to exorcise, which has pictures to show you how to keep in shape. You'll like her approach.

The journey of morning sickness is also depicted in the 29 cartoons of my other book, *Take Two Crackers and Call Me in the Morning! A Real-Life Guide for Surviving Morning Sickness*, which is available in English and in Spanish from (no joke) the Grinnen-Barrett Publishing Company. The book is also carried by amazon.com. Check in with my Web site from time to time (ww.morningsickness.net) and you'll find tidbits of what's new in morning-sickness management. I'll be reporting on new studies, new remedies, and updating the "Queasy Questions" section, which has questions generated by women like you.

GETTING EVEN

One way to purge nasty negative emotions is by using "food voodoo." This little game may sound primitive, but it works well to dissipate anger. You can use any sort of food, but crunchy ones work best. Take a few carrot sticks or celery stalks and pretend they're the legs or arms of the person you're angry with. Bite down hard and work for the loudest noise possible. With every crunch, say to yourself, "There, I got even and now I feel better!" Round raw vegetables, such as radishes, florets of cauliflower, and mushrooms make nice food voodoo heads. Gingerbread men are a good choice as well, for obvious reasons.

Getting rid of stress this way can help relax the muscles in your gastrointestinal tract, improving digestion. When you play food voodoo, you tend to eat foods with high fiber and high water contents, which helps prevent constipation. There's some evidence that chemical compounds in ginger work to stimulate the appetite and calm the gastrointestinal tract, so munching gingerbread men may bring a double benefit. Admittedly, the amount of ginger in gingerbread or ginger cookies can be variable. No one knows for sure what amount is helpful in quelling nausea, but eating can often help reduce nausea.

You may not experience all of these emotions, but just knowing that others have trod the same path should give you some comfort, a sense of sisterhood, and optimism. Negative emotions often grow more powerful when you keep them to yourself; sharing your troubles can divide your worry and lower your stress. Do your best to find someone you can talk with regularly.

DEALING WITH STUPID THINGS PEOPLE SAY

People who know that you have morning sickness often ask how you're feeling. Some genuinely want to know; others come across as armchair quarterbacks. Expect a few to say something crude, stupid, or insensitive. You don't need to answer truthfully or answer at all if it's likely to prolong a conversation you'd prefer not to have. A quick comment or a smile may be all you can muster while struggling to maintain equilibrium. It may help to be prepared for certain comments.

Some people ask the standard questions but don't really want an honest answer. A typical comment is "But you look pretty good." Of course, when quiet nausea turns into a case of dry heaves or vomiting, fewer people want to continue the conversation or hang around and try to help.

Some people like to compare miseries. "Let me tell you how sick my sister Mary was. But she'd get up and drive 50 miles one way to work anyway!"

Some people seem to want to rub it in out of jealousy. This might come from friends or relatives who've been trying for years to become pregnant and have failed. You might hear: "But you should be so happy you're pregnant!"

Some people simply want to keep up on the local gossip. "So, June, you've lost so much weight, what do you weigh now? Isn't that bad for the baby? What is your doctor doing about it?"

Some people seem to try to make you feel guilty. "I don't know anybody else who can't eat or refuses to eat! Just eat! After all, this is going to be a grandchild of mine, and this business has to stop!" It might help to understand that this type of comment really says, "I'm worried about you, and I've never seen you sick. I don't know what to do."

Many pregnant women feel compelled to respond when someone asks, "How are you?" The real answer may be, "miserable," but most women figure the questioner probably wants to hear the brave but bland "I'm really fine." Women are somehow expected to bear up admirably, because "after all, it's only pregnancy!" Many women also want to avoid sounding wimpy and don't care to relive every private agony.

You can reacquaint folks with the sensation of queasiness by encouraging them to see an OmniMax theater performance of *To Fly*. Although the cinematography is spectacular, the rapid-zoom techniques make a good percentage of the audience moderately nauseated. This experience was one I will not easily forget!

Dr. Shari Munch, an assistant professor at Rutgers University, studied women with really bad morning sickness—hyperemesis, in fact—and hits the nail on the head. She says there is a pattern pertaining to the perception that pregnancy is not an illness; pregnant women are not ill women. She goes on to report that although this may be a healthy attitude in general, it places an undue burden on women who suffer with hyperemesis. Her concern, which is a valid one, is that as more women with hyperemesis receive medical therapy at home rather than being hospitalized, their contact with providers and others will be reduced.

You'll probably have a good dozen people ask, "did you eat crackers?" That's the classic one! One woman got so irritated with people asking that, her response was "HELL NO! I like being sick! Try it sometime yourself!" She said she sort of felt bad later about saying that, but the look on the other person's face was worth the shock value.

Chapter 8

A Nutrition Primer

ELENA

An efficient, precise librarian at a major university, Elena spent the majority of both of her pregnancies in the hospital or on her couch. Starting off at a petite 5 feet, 3 inches and 112 pounds, she lost 9 pounds in her first pregnancy. She regained the lost weight 10 months after the pregnancy was over.

Getting pregnant again was not in Elena's immediate plan, because she felt she had not recovered from her first "motherhood" ordeal. However, Elena discovered her unplanned second pregnancy one day while she was changing her daughter's diaper: She became instantly ill. By the following week, she was unable to function in her job, noting that the smell of musty books and manuscripts "made [her] continually nauseous and if [she] wasn't gagging or retching, then [she'd] be vomiting."

Hospitalized on a high-risk pregnancy unit, she made little improvement, except that "the moldy smell was gone." Her nurses, nutritionist, and doctors all tried to coax her to eat, but without success. She finally refused to hear about or talk about food, because the mere mention of it was unsettling. She noted that certain sights added to her queasiness, such as the busy necktie her doctor wore. Noises became more acute than usual, and, interestingly, she found that she drooled more than usual when she was in a noisy environment.

When she finally began to eat, she learned self-hypnosis to "try to keep the food down." She noted that "the minute [her] baby was delivered, [she] could eat!" She asked for and received two roast beef dinners, which she ate: "I told them one was for my husband, but I just knew I was going to be able to chow it right down—and I did!"

I met this librarian as I was digging for historical medical books at the medical library. Once she knew what I was attempting to research, of course, we got into her stories. We talked about the problem of nutrition during morning sickness.

Many salient points about nutrition and pregnancy were evolving in a verse I'd been working on for a pregnancy and parenting newspaper just weeks before. Elena wanted to give it to her cousin Viv, who was contemplating pregnancy. Of course, Elena's cousin was dreadfully worried about having a hyperemesis pregnancy because she was related! Cousin Viv, having spent a year in Japan, knew that Japanese women also had bad morning sickness. A woman in the family she lived with had had it, and they had a special word for it: *Tsuwari*. Viv wanted to max out her nutrition in advance, just in case. She knew two affected women on opposite sides of the globe. She started working on her pregnancy diet.

Keeping this little nutrition reminder on your refrigerator might also help you make smart choices when you have the opportunity.

A Mother's D.I.E.T.(c)
Planning motherhood? It's the best time to explore
the foods and nutrients in the basic four.

Skimmed milk and yogurt with calcium abound.
Don't forget riboflavin, here it is found.

Fresh fruits and juices deliver vitamin C,
some roughage and folate—take it from me.

Green, red, and yellow veggies add a lot to a meal,
loaded with antioxidant vitamins. Such a good deal!

Whole-grain products are nutrient dense.
To include eight daily makes loads of sense.

Lean protein and soy keep the body intact—
critical for life, now that is a fact.

The "extra" category is familiar to all—
the fats and oils, a diet downfall!

This is the group that gets us in trouble.
As far as calories, they provide *double*.

Protein and carb per gram are four.
Fats give us nine—quite a bit more.

Omega 3s are the good fats to partake;
critical for neurons—better brains they make!

Bad fats are tricky since quiet damage they do.
Besides making us chubby, it's free radicals they spew!

Free radicals are enemies in the zest for life,
causing diseases and pain, aggro, and strife!

These are the facts to help us decide
what we should eat or just push aside.

Your baby must eat—remember that line,
as you pull up your chair and sit down to dine.

Don't think of D.I.E.T. in a negative way.
It's a guide to good health: Start today!

(D.I.E.T. is an acronym for *develop intelligent eating techniques*. This
topic will be discussed in greater detail later in this chapter.)

If you're going through morning sickness, it's critical that you maintain the best nutrition you can manage, which is often easier said than done. Sometimes just keeping down any old calorie is a formidable challenge.

This chapter explains the roles of the macronutrients (which provide energy): carbohydrates, proteins, and fats. The more you understand about the way these elements function, the easier it will be for you to make sound decisions about nutrition while you're enduring morning sickness. This chapter will also touch on some events that might come between your fork and digestive tract!

THE BASICS OF NUTRITION

CARBOHYDRATES

Carbohydrates—grains, cereals, fruits, and vegetables—provide various forms of energy, both quick and sustained. Quick energy comes from simple carbohydrates, or sugars (in cookies and candy, for example), which are rapidly digested. Sustained energy comes from the complex carbohydrates, which are more slowly digested. The body can store a limited amount of carbohydrate—about 400 calories worth of energy—in the liver, in the form of glycogen. Muscles also store a small amount of glycogen, which is rapidly used up with activity. However, if more carbohydrate calories are taken in than are needed, the body will store this extra energy as fat. During times of limited intake, fat breakdown will provide calories or energy for the body to burn. Inherent in whole-grain carbohydrates are some of the key B vitamins that are vital for energy metabolism and magnesium. Refined carbohydrates, especially white flour, have lost these nutrients in processing and they have to be added back. Sugar, another carbohydrate, has no vitamins and minerals but does provide calories.

PROTEIN

Meat, fish, cheese, eggs, legumes, and tofu are protein foods. A certain amount of the protein foods you consume are used to keep muscles intact. During pregnancy, protein supports the growth of the new fetus as well as supplying the needs of the mother. Many of the body's enzymes and hormones are made of amino acids, which come from the breakdown of protein. When more protein is eaten than needed, the surplus is stored as fat.

Of the three components of food—carbohydrates, protein, and fat—protein requires the most water to process, because the body must rid itself of excess nitrogen, an element found almost exclusively in proteins. Nitrogen is eliminated from the body mainly in the urine. Many protein foods have a relatively low water content. If you eat a high-protein diet, make sure you have an adequate fluid intake.

A study was done in which pregnant and breast-feeding rats were fed soy's active ingredient, genistein, which has a chemical structure similar to estrogen. The male offspring produced in this study had lower testosterone levels and smaller sexual organs. However, the amount of genistein fed to the mother rats was astronomical compared to what pregnant women eat. (Studying the effects that a mega dose of genistein would have on female rat pups would be interesting.) If eating tofu and drinking soy milk were truly likely to produce the same results for a human pregnancy, I would be expecting front page news from the FDA, ACOG, the March of

Dimes, and other watchdog organizations. Obviously, the rats were fed supplements and not real human food.

FATS AND FATS

Getting away from dietary fat is difficult. Fats are ubiquitous—just about everywhere—except in fruits and vegetables. All fats provide 9 calories per gram; however, some are considered healthier than others. Fats come in a few varieties: saturated and polyunsaturated fats, trans fats, monounsaturated fats, omega 6s, and omega 3s.

The saturated fats—found in fatty meats, butter, eggs, cheese, and whole-milk products raise low-density lipoproteins (LDLs). LDLs are the lousy cholesterol molecules. Saturated fats should be avoided. Besides affecting LDLs, saturated fats may increase blood pressure and increase the risk of blood clots.

As you read in Chapter 3, "Why Do We Get Morning Sickness," a research group looked at the role of saturated fats and the risk of severe morning sickness. The study found that the women with more severe cases of nausea and vomiting during their pregnancy (hyperemesis gravidarum) had had higher saturated fat intakes in the year before their pregnancy. Granted, you can't go back and undo your diet from last year if you're sick now, but for a future pregnancy this is an area for you to consider changing.

Trans fat—the new bad guy on the dietary block—currently is not listed on food product labels but will be by January 1, 2006. Trans fats are found in most margarines, shortenings, deep-fat-fried foods, and commercial pastries and snack foods. These fats lower high-density lipoproteins (HDLs), which are healthy molecules, and raise LDL levels.

Monounsaturated fats are found in plant-based products— olive oil, canola oil, and special safflower and sunflower oils known as high oleic oils. The monos, as they are called, may raise HDLs, lower LDLs, lower blood pressure, and decrease the rate at which LDLs perform metabolic damage.

Although omega-6 fats are found in plant foods, too much of these is bad news. (I think of omega 6s as the deep six—6 feet under!) These are found in corn, safflower, and sunflower oils. We get too many of these.

Omega-3 fats are the good fats. I like to think of these as the trinity fats—or saving-life fats. We don't get enough of the omega 3s, and that's a problem. Researchers are looking at the ratio of omega 6s to 3s for health promotion. Omega-3 fats can be found in fish oil, canola oil, and flaxseed oil as well as in fatty fish and flaxseeds. Omega 3s increase HDLs, lower LDLs, lower blood pressure, and reduce the risk of blood clots.

Here are some books that will help you incorporate healthier eating into your life easily, while explaining nutrition clearly: *The Omega Diet: The Life-Saving Nutritional Program Based on the Diet of the Island of Crete*, *The Whole Foods Market Cookbook*, and *Becoming Vegan: The Complete Guide to Adopting a Healthy Plant-Based Diet*.

CALORIES AND KETONES

Problems begin when a pregnant woman is unable to ingest the daily calories she requires. First, her body uses up glycogen, a stored form of carbohydrate. Then it begins to use stored fat for energy, and next it uses muscle. This is what normally happens when you go on a weight-loss diet. One difference is that on a moderate weight-loss diet, the planned calorie deficit each day is probably only a few hundred calories. But severe nausea and vomiting are not planned, and the resulting calorie deficit is often beyond your control.

Assume for a moment that the average pregnant woman in her first trimester needs to consume 1,700 to 2,200 calories a day, depending on height, prepregnancy body size, and general activity. (Recommended Dietary Intakes, the RDIs, add 300 calories per day for pregnancy at the beginning of the second trimester. This assumes, of course, that there are no unusual situations, such as weight loss caused by morning sickness.) When a pregnant woman is unable to take in (and keep down) the required maintenance calories, her body has no choice but to burn (metabolize) fat and muscle to make energy.

One of the by-products of burning fat, or fat metabolism, is the production of ketones (pronounced "key tones"), which are a type of organic acid that the body produces (keto-acids). Ketones give your breath a peculiar, fruity smell, and they can be one of the factors responsible for the bad taste in the mouth that many pregnant women have. Ketones are a red flag that the body is in starvation mode and in some state of nutritional compromise. The body tries to get rid of ketones by exhaling them or passing them out through the urine. Doctors usually check for urine ketones and take action before critical levels accumulate in the blood. If the body is also becoming dehydrated, the ketone concentration in the blood can be even higher. Another reported effect from high levels of ketones is nausea. Ketones can be eliminated fairly quickly by eating small amounts of carbohydrates regularly.

THE DANGERS OF DEHYDRATION

Water is the nutrient most critical to life. When your fluid consumption doesn't satisfy your body's needs because nausea prevents you from eating and drinking, or because you keep vomiting, dehydration is often the consequence. Because dehydration has an immediate effect on all body functions, it calls for medical intervention—possibly a trip to an emergency room for outpatient fluid therapy.

Dehydration is a serious problem because it can affect your blood pressure. If your blood pressure gets too low, it can cause fainting, low urine output, and reduced nutrient supplies for the fetus; all of which are potentially harmful. If you're suffering from these symptoms, a hospital stay may be necessary (see Chapter 11). Chronic dehydration will eventually affect how much amniotic fluid is produced.

If vomiting becomes more severe, vital minerals (called electrolytes) are lost, along with gastrointestinal fluids. The major electrolytes are potassium, sodium, phosphorous, magnesium, and chloride. Each plays an important role in body functions. Minerals help muscles to contract and relax, especially the muscles of the heart, which pump blood to all parts of the body. Lowered levels of potassium, magnesium, and sodium can result in weaker heart contractions or irregular heartbeats. Low levels of phosphorous affect respiratory muscle function and energy metabolism. When body fluid is lost, the volume of blood that the heart has to pump is also reduced.

BONE HEALTH

Inactivity and bone health have been investigated in pregnant women put on bed rest for pregnancy complications. Because pressure is not exerted on the ends of long bones when you are at bed rest, calcium is released. What's even scarier is that the amount of calcium released from the skeleton is unrelated to dietary intake.

I've talked to many morning sickness sufferers who have been told by their doctors that their bones are 30 years older than they are. Bone density loss is a real liability of morning sickness and the accompanying malnutrition. Osteopenia, or reduced bone mass, is a problem when a woman's prepregnancy diet was low in calcium. If a less-than-nutritious pregegancy routine is followed by a bad case of morning sickness, and a healthy pregnancy diet is not achievable, osteopenia often results.

One case in the medical literature is particularly striking. A group of bone specialists in Boston cared for a woman with a severe bone loss. This woman, an obstetric nurse, had a history of ankylosing spondylitis, had bad morning sickness, and lost 10 pounds in her first trimester. Her overall pregnancy weight gain was 19 pounds over her starting weight. That's about 75 percent of the normal expected weight gain. Because of her history of ankylosing spondylitis, she lost 4 inches of height as well!

There are a few other case reports about postpartum bone loss but decreased intake during pregnancy wasn't noted in these cases. It's hard to imagine that if the diet was optimal in pregnancy and before, these problems would show up only in the postpartum period. I suspect these results that show problems with intake during the pregnancies are most likely related to morning sickness.

Calcium is mobilized from the bones, and the amount lost is unrelated to the amount taken in with the diet. Therefore, it is important to replace calcium that is lost. Granted, during the hard days of nausea and vomiting, eating enough calcium-rich dairy products and leafy greens is going to be hard. Certain foods from the meat, dairy, and fruit and vegetables groups are rich in calcium. If you can't get in your daily allowance, calcium candy chews might help (e.g., Viactiv and Calcium Chews). Flavors are chocolate, caramel, and fruit. Calorie content might vary, but each is about 20 to 30 calories and has 300 to 500 milligrams of calcium per chew. At any rate, if you spent a good part of your pregnancy horizontal, you'll want to be sure to talk to your doctor about a postpartum bone-density evaluation. Catching reduced bone mass as early as possible will give you a chance to do some nutrititional catch-up. We talked about this in an earlier chapter, but it's important to be reminded of this serious morning-sickness-related problem.

It's important to talk to your doctor about your prepregnancy calcium intake. Calcium is an important component for your developing baby. If your intake is poor, it comes out of your hide, not the baby's! I recommend postpartum bone density evaluations to be sure any insult to the bones is taken care of immediately. By all means, ask your doctor for a referral to a Registered Dietitian (R.D.) who has experience with pregnancy problems. A group of specialized R.D.s belong to the Women in Reproductive Nutrition Practice group of the American Dietetic Association. Call (800) 877-1600 and ask for the list.

MUSCLE LOSS AND MORNING SICKNESS

Muscle is lost as well as calcium. Whether you are in a hospital bed or doing the couch potato routine at home, you will experience muscle loss. An astonishing 25 to 30 percent of muscle volume loss can occur with a 5-week stint in bed! Exercising muscles regularly can help reduce muscle loss. Ask for a referral to a registered physical therapist.

YOUR WEIGHT AND MORNING SICKNESS

A net weight loss does not always accompany morning sickness. Although many women who aren't able to eat regularly lose a few real and fluid pounds, not all do, for the following reasons:

1. The pregnancy hormones, especially estrogen, help the body retain fluid. Because body fluid is part of body mass, any gain or loss can make a difference when you get onto the scale. The pregnancy hormones also slow down the rate at which food goes through the body; more calories are thought to be absorbed when this occurs.

2. If weight declines slowly, the body sometimes readjusts its basal metabolic rate, becoming more efficient and using fewer calories— perhaps by lowering the body temperature a fraction, or by reducing the number of respirations or heartbeats in a given period. In addition, when you feel ill, you automatically reduce your physical activity, which saves calories. Just as a point of reference, the number of calories needed to maintain the weight of a healthy adult is about 1 to 1.25 per minute, barring exercise or extraordinary activity. This is the basal metabolic rate or the number of calories it takes to operate the body at rest. This works out to be about 1,440 calories for the average woman, who is 5 feet, 5 inches tall and 120 pounds. Dietitians add another 25 percent for usual activities, which in this example would work out to 360 calories, making the maintenance total about 1,800 calories a day.

   Putting calories into perspective, a slice of toast, about 70 calories, will provide the average woman with enough fuel to operate metabolically for about 1 hour. For the father of the baby, an average, physically fit man weighing approximately

180 pounds, this same slice of toast will probably be used up in less than 40 minutes. The reason for the difference is that most men have more muscle and less fat mass than most women, and muscles use more energy than fat mass uses.

3. You may eat more during your good periods than you realize. A switch from three cans of diet soda a day to five cans of regular soda means 800 calories, whereas the diet soda's caloric contribution would have been zero, or perhaps 40 percent of a day's caloric requirement. Fifteen soda crackers could mean about 280 calories, or almost one-seventh of the average daily requirement of 2,000 calories.

Your perception that you're starving may be amplified because your food choices are often narrowed. The food suggestions generally given to sick women usually stick to the bland and white or tan foods. These suggestions come from families as well as health-care providers and have been handed down through the years as remedies that work for everyone.

4. Fluid losses with vomiting make weight loss difficult to assess from day to day. The time of day, the scale used, and the absence or presence of bowel movements can also affect the weight measurement.

Because everyone is concerned with weight changes, the smallest downward trend can spark panic, which may be a bit premature. A weight monitoring chart is provided in Appendix A of this book to help you plot the changes during your pregnancy.

Despite the apparent contradiction, many women achieve very high weight peaks in their pregnancies because of nausea and vomiting. Many find that eating something—anything—all the time makes them feel better, or at least "less horrible."

What Is Expected Weight Gain?

Weight loss in pregnancy is not anticipated; rather, there is supposed to be a certain percentage of weight gain (see the chart in Appendix A for the expected weight gain based on prepregnancy weight). Detecting malnutrition in pregnant women is crucial to their health as well as to the health of their babies. Women with low weight gains are more susceptible to problems with postpartum depression, and they have fewer energy reserves. In addition, weight loss in pregnancy predisposes women to have babies that are small for gestational age (SGA babies).

To evaluate the degree of malnutrition, the amount of actual gain (or loss) needs to be compared to the expected weight gain. It makes sense to add the lack of weight gain to the actual weight loss to measure the gross loss in weight during pregnancy. (As of the writing of this book, there is no consensus in clinical practice on how to interpret a deficit in expected weight gain because no one has really addressed it.) For example, one woman ended her pregnancy 20 pounds heavier than her prepregnancy weight (that is, her net weight gain was 20 pounds). However, 20 pounds was only 60 percent of her expected weight gain (so she had a net deficit of about 13 pounds compared to her expected weight gain).

MOVING ON: THE IMPORTANCE OF D.I.E.T.

Once the nausea and vomiting have passed, it's time to try to nutritious foods again. If you're to stay healthy, you need to D.I.E.T., which, again, stands for develop intelligent eating techniques. Schedule an appointment with a registered dietitian (R.D.) for a complete nutritional assessment. An R.D. will evaluate the nutrient contribution of the foods you usually eat. Certain foods may remain problematic for you. If you can't tolerate milk, for example, your diet may be low in calcium, as well as in the vitamin riboflavin. If you got sick on some of your favorite healthy foods, you might continue to avoid them after all your morning sickness is over. This is a sort of scape-goating. Sometimes it takes a long time to reaccept and reincorporate particular foods back into the diet. The R.D. will help find alternative ways to provide missing nutrients to your diet and will discuss with you better or new ways to prepare food.

Only after a careful analysis of your usual intake will the R.D. suggest supplemental vitamins and minerals. One reason for is that some nutrients (calcium, for example) are better absorbed from foods than from pills. I've cared for a number of women who have had accelerated bone loss because of a hard pregnancy, and a very limited calcium intake. If your daily intake was virtually nonexistent before you got pregnant and you couldn't consume 4 servings of dairy a day for the majority of your pregnancy or take calcium supplements, be sure you mention it to you doctor. It is better to find out now about bone loss and begin treatment than to find out in 20 years that your bones look like a block of Swiss cheese.

Another nutrient to pay attention to is iron. Taking iron supplements causes constipation for the majority of women, but I've counseled a few (5 to 10 percent) for whom the iron seemed to give them the opposite problem. Delicate relationships exist among the various nutrients; they are easily disturbed if the dose of any supplement is excessive, or over 100 percent of the RDIs. A carefully selected daily diet can supply many of nutrients needed for a healthy pregnancy.

Try to eat according to this general daily-minimum guide:

4 servings from the dairy group

10 or more servings from the fruit and vegetable groups

6–8 servings from the whole-grains and breads groups

2 servings (each 3 ounces) from the protein, fish, poultry, and lean-meat group (more emphasis on fish because of its positive health contributions)

3 to 4 teaspoons fat (emphasis on the polyunsaturated and monounsaturated fats, no trans fat—this means more canola oils and olive oils and less butter, lard, and hydrogenated fats)

No one food contains all the nutrients you need when you're pregnant, so variety is the word. Check out the list of nutrients that fall into each food grouping in the following list, and the need for a sensible balance will become obvious. Consider buying organic foods, even though they are somewhat more expensive. Fewer pesticides and insecticides have been used on them, and no synthetic fertilizers have been used. There are regulations for U.S. growers who claim products are organic. (See the discussion on organic foods in the appendix.)

MEAT AND PROTEIN GROUP

Fish (Eat smaller fish, because they have less exposure to mercury. Keep in touch with your local fish advisory service about mercury levels.)

Poultry

Beef (Choose lean animal protein products which means cut off any white fat before you cook your item. If you can blot the

surface with a paper napkin, you can remove some additional fat.)
Pork
Lamb
Eggs (Eggs can be a source of omega-3 fatty acids if the hens producing them were fed omega-3 meal.)
Low-fat cheeses
Legumes
Tofu
Nuts

The calories, or energy, provided by these foods come from complete protein and, in many cases, from hidden fat. Meats should be lean, with fat trimmed off. Don't eat raw or undercooked meat, chicken, or fish! Food poisoning, such as listeria, has been positively associated with stillbirths. Soft cheese and deli meats are items that have been implicated in listeria food poisoning. Pregnancy reduces a woman's immune status, which is why, as a group, pregnant women are more at risk for picking up bad bugs.

Foods in this group contain the following vitamins and minerals:

Thiamin (vitamin B_1)
Riboflavin (vitamin B_2)
Niacin
Vitamin B_6
Vitamin A
Vitamin D
Vitamin K
Calcium
Chloride

Cobalt
Phosphorus
Sodium
Zinc
Copper
Iodine
Iron
Biotin
Pantothenic acid
Folic acid (or folate)
Vitamin B_{12}
Molybdenum
Potassium
Magnesium
Sulfur

Dairy Group

Low-fat and skim milk
Low-fat yogurt
Low-fat cottage cheese
Ice milk
Low-fat cheeses

Calories, or energy, in this group come from complete protein, some fat, and some carbohydrate.

The following vitamins and minerals are found in dairy food:

Thiamin (vitamin B_1)
Riboflavin (vitamin B_2)

Vitamin A
Vitamin D
Calcium
Chloride
Phosphorus
Sodium
Sulfur
Magnesium
Biotin
Vitamin B_{12}
Potassium
Zinc
Selenium

FRUIT AND VEGETABLE GROUP

The more colorful your choice of fruit or vegetable, the more phytonutrients it contains!

Fruits and Juices

Apple
Apple juice (Generally not a good source of vitamins—take a peek at the label.)
Orange
Orange juice (If your dairy intake is low, opt for calcium-enriched orange juice.)
Cranberry juice
Banana

Pear

Peach (Always wash this fruit carefully. One research group found very high levels of pesticides in peaches because they get caught in the fuzzy skin.)

Pineapple

Prunes (now called dried plums)

Prune juice

Kiwi

Mango

Guava

Strawberries

Blueberries

Raspberries

Blackberries

Cherries

Grapes (opt for red grapes)

Plums

Apricots

Apricot nectar

Vegetables

Asparagus

Broccoli

Brussels sprouts

Cabbage, red and green

Dandelion greens

Endive

Cauliflower

Carrots

Eggplant

Kale

Mustard greens

Parsnips

Green and yellow beans

Yams

Sweet potatoes

Peas

Potatoes

Tomatoes

Zucchini

Winter squash

Pumpkins

In the fruit and vegetable group, calories, or energy, come from carbohydrates. These foods contain the following vitamins and minerals:

Riboflavin (vitamin B_2)

Niacin

Vitamin A

Vitamin E

Vitamin K

Calcium

Phosphorus

Potassium

Copper

Iron

Magnesium

Molybdenum

Folic acid

Ascorbic acid

Fiber

Manganese

BREADS, CEREALS, AND STARCHY VEGETABLES GROUP

Rice (opt for brown rice)

Pasta (try whole-wheat pasta products)

Noodles

Potatoes

Corn

Squash (winter type)

Wheat, rye, oatmeal, and white bread

Crackers

Rolls (opt for products with whole grains, which are more nutritious.)

Whole-grain cooked cereal

Ready-to-eat dry cereal (try the high-fiber soy products)

Popcorn (unbuttered)

Muffins (With super-sizing, many muffins are now 6 ounces, about the size of a coffee cup; 10 years ago, the average muffin was slightly smaller than a woman's fist, about 3 ounces.

Tabbouleh (made from cracked bulgur wheat)

Bread/cereal group calories, or energy, come from complex carbohydrates and incomplete protein. They provide the following vitamins and minerals:

Thiamin (vitamin B_2)

Niacin

Vitamin B_6

Selenium

Phosphorus

Sulfur

Zinc

Copper

Iron

Magnesium

Manganese

Molybdenum

Pantothenic acid

Biotin

Potassium

Fiber

Chromium

Selenium

FATS

Current nutrition research suggests that the amount of fat in the overall daily diet should be kept between 30 to 40 percent of total calories. There are three general types of fats to consider: polyunsaturated, monounsaturated, and saturated.

The amount of saturated fat in food seems to be correlated most strongly with major disease, which is why nutritionists suggest eating less than 10 percent of your total daily calories from this type. Saturated fats are generally solid at room temperature and are found in meats, cheeses, and milk products, in addition to palm-kernel and coconut oils. Monounsaturated oils include flaxseed, olive, and canola. Polyunsaturated oils include corn, safflower, and sunflower. Soon labels will be required to post the amount of trans fats. Trans fats have been found to be positively correlated with disease processes, so you should steer away from them.

If you cook with any of the nut oils (almond, walnut, pecan, peanut oil) always be sure to let everyone know that you do. With the huge increase in nuts allergies, this is a severe health-risk problem.

RDI NUTRIENTS

Here's a quick review of what each of the nutrients listed in the RDIs does. This is a streamlined version. For more details, consult a book on nutrition or see an R.D.

- Protein helps to keep muscles intact, builds red blood cells, makes antibodies (germ fighters) and maintains the structural parts of the body.
- Carbohydrates provide the body with quick energy. Many nutrients are found in carbohydrate foods.
- Fats provide three essential fatty acids, which keep the skin looking healthy. Getting enough is not generally a problem; getting the *right kind* of fat is the problem. Eat more omega 3s and less omega 6s.
- Vitamin A keeps eyes healthy and keeps the membranes that line the body intact.
- Vitamin C keeps intact the connective tissue (the tissue that holds your blood vessels together and that holds bones to muscles), reduces bruising, and keeps gums strong.

- Vitamin D contains phosphorus and calcium, which keep bones and teeth strong.
- Vitamin K helps blood clot effectively and is important in bone health.
- Vitamin E protects cells from oxidation (a process that destroys them).
- Thiamin (also known as vitamin B_1) releases energy from carbohydrate foods and aids in proper functioning of the heart, gastrointestinal tract, and nervous system.
- Riboflavin (also known as vitamin B_2) releases energy from carbohydrates, proteins, and fats and makes red blood cells.
- Niacin releases energy from carbohydrates; it also contributes to fat synthesis and metabolism.
- Vitamin B_6 is important in the metabolism of carbohydrates, fats, and protein; proper functioning of the central nervous system; and other activities.
- Vitamin B_{12} is important for the normal functioning of the gastrointestinal tract, bone marrow (red blood cell production), and nervous system as well as for growth. It is involved in the formation of myelin, the coating around the nerves, and in the metabolism of carbohydrates, proteins, and fat. Vitamin B_{12} prevents serious anemia.
- Biotin is necessary for many enzyme systems in the body.
- Pantothenic acid is part of the enzyme systems. It is important for the proper metabolism of carbohydrates, proteins, and fats.
- Folic acid is necessary for the production of DNA and the functioning of two amino acids. Folic acid is also essential for the formation of both white and red blood cells. It is

critical for preventing neutral tube defects—a fetal development problem.

- Choline is important for the proper metabolism of fats.
- Calcium is important for strong bones and teeth, muscle and heart contractions, and blood clotting.
- Phosphorus works with calcium and vitamin D to make strong bones and teeth and aids many metabolic reactions in the body.
- Magnesium is used for many energy reactions, proper blood clotting, and muscular contractions—notably for muscle relaxation. Magnesium has important roles in cardiovascular disease, diabetes, migraine management, and osteoporosis prevention. The RDI in pregnancy is 400 milligrams per day.
- Iron carries oxygen to all cells in the body and is part of many enzyme systems.
- Zinc is part of many enzyme systems in the body and is critical for immune function maintenance.
- Iodine is a thyroid hormone, which regulate the body's metabolism.
- Selenium protects other nutrients.
- Copper is important in many enzyme systems and in preventing anemia.
- Manganese is important in enzyme systems for proper reproduction, growth, and bone and cartilage function as well as for glucose metabolism.
- Fluoride strengthens bones and teeth.
- Chromium is important for proper glucose metabolism.
- Molybdenum is important in many enzyme systems.

- Sodium is important in the maintenance of fluid balance in the body.
- Potassium is important for nerve functioning, skeletal and cardiac muscle contractions, and maintaining blood pressure.
- Chloride is essential for maintaining fluid and electrolyte balance.

If you take vitamins and minerals, be sure not to take over 100 percent of any unless you have been specially advised to do so. More is not necessarily better! Some vitamins and minerals can accumulate in your body and become toxic. Excessively high levels of vitamin A can cause birth defects, for example. If you take prescription medication, there might be requirements for extra vitamins and minerals. One example of this is Dilantin, which is used for seizure control and affects folic acid metabolism.

Commonly prescribed antacids change the pH or the acidity of your stomach. Antacids make your stomach less acidic, and that change can decrease the absorption of calcium, iron, magnesium, and zinc. Sometimes eating more slowly, chewing well, and eating six to seven smaller meals a day can obviate the need to take antacids.

QUICK NUTRIENT CALCULATOR

Item	Amount	Calories	Protein (in grams)
Liquids			
Club soda	12 oz	0	0
Tonic water	12 oz	120	0
Ginger ale	12 oz	115	0
Cola	12 oz	140	0

Item	Amount	Calories	Protein (in grams)
Milk, skim	8 oz	80	8
Milk, low-fat	8 oz	100	8
Milk, whole	8 oz	150	8
Apple juice	4 oz	60	0
Lemonade	8 oz	70	0
Cocoa	8 oz	220	9
Smoothies (see recipes)	8oz	varies	varies
Starches			
Cream of wheat	1/2 cup	70	2
Cold cereal	1/2 cup	75	2
Toast	1 slice	75	2
Rice cake	1 (3 in.)	50	1
English muffin	1 whole	150	4
Corn muffin	1 small	145	3
Mashed potatoes	1/2 cup	75	2
Noodles	1/2 cup	100	2
Rice	1/2 cup	100	3
French fries	1 oz	150	2
Popcorn	1 oz	140	2
Pretzels	1 oz	95	2
Pancakes, 2	3-in. dia.	120	4
Saltines	6	70	2
Vegetables			
Squash	1/2 cup	40	1
Creamed corn	1/2 cup	80	2
Green beans	1/2 cup	30	1
Carrots, raw	1/2 cup	25	1
Tomato	1 whole	30	1
Broccoli	1/2 cup	30	1
Mixed salad	2 cups	50	1
Desserts			
Tapioca	1/2 cup	110	4

Custard	1/2 cup	150	7
Ice cream	1/2 cup	150	3
Gelatin	1/2 cup	80	1
Popsicle	3 oz	70	0
Sherbet	1/2 cup	120	3
Angel-food cake	1/12th	90	2
Nuts	1 oz	175	6
Soups and Entrees			
Chicken rice soup	1/2 cup	30	2
Grilled cheese sandwich	1	325	18
Macaroni and cheese	6 oz	200	1
Chicken pot pie	8 oz	450	15
Pizza, cheese	4 oz	320	14
Skinless chicken breast	2 oz	160	14

MAGNESIUM-RICH FOODS

Food	Milligrams
1 medium artichoke	180
1 cup boiled spinach	160
1/2 cup 100% bran cereal	115
1 medium Florida avocado	105
1 medium (3 oz) oat bran muffin	90
1 oz almonds	85
1 oz dry roasted cashews	75
1/2 cup edamame (soybeans)	75
1 cup boiled lentils	70
1/2 cup wheat germ	70
1/2 cup cooked black beans	60
1 medium baked potato with skin	55
2 tablespoons peanut butter	50
28 dry roasted peanuts	50

2 slices whole-wheat bread	50
1/2 cup cooked brown rice	50
1 cup cooked beets	40
1 cup cooked broccoli	40
1 oz sunflower seeds	40
1 medium banana	35

Chapter 9

Managing Morning Sickness with Food

ISABELLE

A seemingly happily married woman with three children and a magnificently adoring and financially successful husband, stunning Isabelle at 39 looked as if nothing had ever gone awry in her life—she looked in her mid 20s at most!

She'd been sick with her first pregnancy at age 26. She figured it was normal—that's what the books said. She had lost 8 pounds by week 20 and eventually had delivered at 20 pounds over her prepregnancy weight. She thought it couldn't happen with her second pregnancy, but it did. Her morning sickness was not really outrageous. It was after her third pregnancy—13 years later—that she reported the many details of her capricious morning sickness and how worn out she really was.

She disclosed her true stress level during a session with a social worker. She was adopted and wondered what her birth mother had been like. She thought she had some vague memories but was not sure whether they were real or were just images she had made up over time. Her adoptive parents—financially well-endowed—were delighted to receive Isabelle as an answer to their prayers. They were ill at ease when she started asking real and serious questions about her biological parents at age 12.

It was during this third pregnancy that she had to pull off to the side of the road to vomit and a police cruiser pulled up behind her car with its lights flashing to ask why she was throwing up. She was humiliated beyond words. Obviously this seasoned veteran officer had never had a wife with morning sickness. The officer decided that she was not intoxicated and eventually drove away.

One of the first things she noted was a constant weird taste in her mouth—*metallic* is the best word she could come up with to describe it—and she became very concerned about the freshness of her breath. Like other women, she found the breath of other people difficult to endure. She noted that, oddly, she felt more at ease if her stomach seemed empty rather than full. Morning sickness anorexia would sort of describe how she felt. However, she did force herself to eat and gain the appropriate 30 pounds during her pregnancy.

In contrast to her two previous pregnancies, this time she wanted food after she vomited. She loved the theory of "radar nose" and learned that the slightest scent could set off queasiness. Her description was perfect: She felt like a volcano ready to fire up and out. This time around, she found that Di-Gel antacid tablets worked best for her heartburn. Her tactile senses were escalated as well. Pressure on her navel created nausea, but she found a solution. She made a small pad of gauze and put it over her navel with surgical tape.

After eating, Isabelle found that lying on her right side propped up by two pillows was helpful. The nausea and vomiting lasted her whole pregnancy, except for a short respite in the second trimester. At that time, she craved strong, spicy foods. Tacos, nachos, dips, chips, BBQ ribs, onion rings, and stuffed clams were items her husband, Mark, learned to procure "yesterday." Isabelle also gravitated to cinnamon, ginger, almond, nutmeg, and fennel seeds as stomach settlers. She ate popcorn and bacon, lettuce, and tomato sandwiches for a while, but once they lost their effect, they were off the menu for the duration.

The only two foods that Isabelle could always tolerate, through all three pregnancies, were cold lobster salad and shrimp salad smothered in lemon juice. Beef and pork were definitely out—previously her favorite grilled dinner meals.

She also noted that fatigue and extremes of temperature set her off. She always got sick whenever she began to shiver or sweat. Because her rest was disturbed often, she had trouble with migraine headaches.

A brief trial of vitamin B_6 proved futile. She switched brands of prenatal vitamins, because the original horse pills she got seemed only to make the nausea worse. She took her folic acid tablets and Ferrous Sequels with freshly squeezed homemade orange juice, which surprisingly did not cause any discomfort. She liked the smell of the oranges. Isabelle said she had developed "exogenous constipation" because there were too many people in her household for too few bathrooms; she endured a failed attempt with Fiber Con, which only caused bloating. She couldn't drink as much water as the product suggested, and that was a problem. Isabelle felt dizzy much of the time, and her doctor commented frequently that her blood pressure was low. Though she felt "green" up to month 9, it all ended with the birth of her third child, a healthy girl.

CAN FOOD HELP?

"Eating something specific" was the most commonly reported strategy to ease nausea according to a study in 1989. Successful types of food were, in descending order, crackers, bread, fruit, cereal, dairy products, sweets, meats, and salty foods.

Digestion, for all intents and purposes, begins in the brain. Thinking about food (even dreaming) starts the digestive juices flowing. The process of chewing breaks down food mechanically at the same time that the enzymes in saliva begin to break down food chemically. The amount of saliva produced varies with the degree of saltiness or tartness and with the texture (smooth or rough) of a specific food. From the stomach, food moves through the gastrointestinal tract, again at varying rates. It is reported that high-fat meals stay in the stomach longer than do starchy, low-fat meals and that liquids empty out faster than do solid meals and saltier foods.

Bile, produced by the gallbladder, is released when fat is part of the diet. Some women with severe morning sickness develop thick bile or "sludge" if their intake of fluids drops abnormally low for long periods; this can contribute to gallbladder disease in pregnancy, because highly concentrated sludge can crystallize into small stones. Sometimes very small amounts of potato chips might help to empty the gallbladder periodically and prevent gallstones from forming.

Food choices are often subconscious, and I believe we intuitively gravitate to the foods and beverages that make us feel comforted. It's important to note that the comfort food of a sick person will probably not be the comfort food of a well person. The care provider sees the woman with morning sickness in a dehydrated or semidehydrated state and naturally wants to encourage the woman to drink more liquids. The woman herself, however, is more inclined to eat solid foods because they reduce the queasiness (however, women may crave liquids to reduce the terrible sensation of thirst). The key to breaking the cycle of nausea and vomiting is to alternate food and liquid in the pattern that brings most comfort to the pregnant woman.

Without being obviously aware of it, most people are ethnocentric and egocentric about the foods they choose to eat. This is part of a concept called *organoleptics*, which really means that people make judgments about food by looking at it and by previous experiences of taste, smell, and texture. Getting people to deviate from their usual daily diets is difficult. Most people don't eat unknown food without a lot of coaxing. Most food is categorized as good or bad or weird, whether healthy or junk, within milliseconds, in my estimation. If the verdict is negative, one is hardpressed to reverse that opinion.

Food gets particular attention when someone is sick and pregnant. If you're sick and pregnant, you may find that everyone who has ever read anything about morning sickness becomes an instant in-your-face expert. You'll undoubtedly be offered dozens of food solutions, mainly "eat crackers," the traditional safe recommendation. For some women, crackers work. For others, a cracker is a trillion miles away from providing relief. Your brain might be asking for some very unusual combinations that other people brand as very bizarre. How others react to your food requests will make a difference whether you pursue it or not. Try not to cave in to someone's adverse reaction to your request.

Having had the benefit of eating and enjoying traditional foods from several different cultures (the Caribbean, South Africa, South American, the Turkish region, eastern Europe, Scandinavian countries, and the Mediterranean region), I might ask the following questions of women from those areas: How you would describe your favorite foods? Are smells and aromas different or are tastes and textures different? Being an ethnic cookbooks collector, I think there are interesting implications to be derived from tracing what seasonings are in ethnic dishes. Also, knowing how food is assembled is important because the aromas generated are different with each food combination.

Putting a corral around changes in taste and smell is incredibly difficult because those two aspects are subjective. And, in my opinion and experience, those two aspects can change rapidly. How and why this happens has not been explored to date.

FIGURING OUT WHAT TO EAT

Ask yourself this question: What food or beverage would ease your nausea? Something salty, sour, bitter, tart, sweet, crunchy/lumpy, soft/smooth, mushy, hard, fruity, wet, dry, bland, spicy, aromatic, earthy, hot, cold, thin, or thick? Generally speaking, these adjectives cover almost all foods and beverages. Interestingly, when you start to think about these characteristics, new lists of foods and beverages emerge. Each, of course, contains varying amounts of nutrients, water, and fiber. Each food or beverage may be successful under certain conditions only, for example, in the absence of other food aromas or at a particular time of day. Only by beginning a systematic search will you unearth possible answers. Keeping a daily food diary can be extremely helpful in discovering your tendencies. Your nutritionist can use such a diary to evaluate your diet and help you manage your weight.

Keeping foods in mind, consider the following questions: Would something salty reduce or aggravate the queasy feelings at this very minute? What food or drink comes to mind at this very moment? If it could be procured instantly, would you eat it? Why or why not? Would something crunchy diminish your nausea? If so, what sort of color or flavor would it have? What sort of food or beverage, however bizarre or atypical of your usual choices, appeals to you at this very moment? (Whether or not it's in season is immaterial. Most foods are available almost year-round at premium prices in specialty stores. It could be well worth a special trip and the extra money if that particular food made you feel like the million-dollar mom you are going to be!) Keep asking these three or four questions until you've gone through all the food characteristic adjectives. You'll be surprised at the number of new foods and beverages that come to mind.

It's not uncommon for a woman first to find something she wants to eat in the salty, sour, bitter, or sweet category. It seems that if you can drive the sensation of thirst away with a food from one of these categories, drinking fluids follows more naturally. Recently, I had remarkable success when I gave one of my hospitalized morning sickness clients several Tootsie Rolls, which were what she requested and could eat and keep down. Several hours later she began drinking adequate fluids, and we broke her cycle of nausea and vomiting.

Another woman, admitted at least five times in her first trimester of pregnancy, found on her fourth admission that sour-cream-and-onion-flavored potato chips were the food that helped her break the cycle. Yet another, having been transferred to us after 1 month on intravenous feeding at another hospital, was eating within 3 days. Among the few changes that accompanied her transfer was an ad lib diet order—we served what she asked for.

And although some hospitals claim to have "hyperemesis diets," we really don't know what those are. There isn't one group of foods that works for everyone! We may never know whether it was this woman's newly acquired habit of beginning her meal by dipping raw carrots and celery sticks into a cup of vinegar, the discontinuation of her intravenous feedings, or a change her medication routine that effected the improvement. Both the patient and her family found it odd that her new ritual of dipping the vegetables in vinegar seemed to help her eat more. After eating about three or four sticks each of raw celery and carrot, she would eat approximately three-quarters of each meal, and she drank at least 1.5 quarts of fluid each day.

I've had much success with lemonade, probably because of its aroma and refreshing tartness. From a nutritional management standpoint, the consequences of eating unconventional foods like those described in the three cases above are minuscule and often short-lived. A queasy pregnant woman who chooses a novel food and can eat it almost at the moment she decides she wants it seems to have a greater likelihood of keeping the food down and keeping nausea and vomiting at bay.

Another woman, who was sent to us on intravenous nutrition, had a numb feeling in her feet, among a few complaints. Changes made were a discontinuation of the intravenous nutrition, adding extra vitamins, and reducing smells. As I recall, many of her friends and relatives sent piles of flowers—some of which were really stinky! I asked her if she found them relaxing and she sort of said, "well . . . there are a *lot* of them! I'm not sure whether the smells are making me sick or not. I know everyone wants me to get better quick!"

After a bit of trial and error of sniffing, we weeded some varieties out—especially Rhubrum lilies—but sent many of the flowers home with her husband. This woman decided to keep a bouquet of peonies. She sniffed one peony petal until it was worn out and then went for another one! When I started to feed her, she asked for mashed potatoes, which I delivered. Going back to check, she reluctantly told me that they didn't work—they were too spicy! I'd heard this particular comment before from another woman on intravenous nutrition but didn't pay much attention to it. One such comment goes into my "interesting" category; two go into my "is this a trend?" file. The two women had much in common, and I began to think that starvation must have altered their senses of taste, particularly regarding bland foods. I thought that this was going to be another one of those nights when I would have to go to the library and start digging. But a call to the kitchen to check what ingredients or additives were in the potatoes revealed that one of the ingredients was white pepper! Apparently, it's more aesthetic to not see pepper in mashed potatoes (I've always used black pepper in my mashed potatoes so never gave it a thought). It was a heads up—some of these ladies have "radar tongue" too! We ordered specially prepared, plain, no-pepper, mashed potatoes, and she could eat it without a problem. This one little piece of the food puzzle was a Perry Mason moment for me!

One reason that some women do not acknowledge the urge for novel foods they really want is that more often than not the foods falls into the junk food category. I've asked many women why they don't eat a junk food, when it appeals to them, to get in some calories, and the overwhelming answer is guilt. Prenatal books cover nutrition and discuss benefits of good dietary habit and rightly so. Some women have poor diets before pregnancy, so filling in the nutritional cracks as soon as possible is really important. That job should have been started before getting pregnant, however.

Many women believe that if they consume anything on the "do not eat" list, the baby will immediately suffer. Although it is true that a pregnancy will benefit by better eating habits, in morning sickness, eating it is a very different game. What's the benefit of eating well, vomiting, and having to take antivomiting medication rather than eating a few junk foods, foregoing medication, and not vomiting? It's a game of trade-offs.

Next ask: When you feel the absolute worst, if any food or drink could be delivered instantaneously, what would it be? Would the likelihood that you'd consume it be higher than average if you could have immediate delivery? Does the urge to eat or drink evaporate while you're waiting for the food or beverage? How many minutes after you make a food request does your desire to eat diminish? What factors besides time are associated with closing of the window of opportunity—noise, motion, a smell?

If you had to prepare the food yourself, did you lose your desire to eat because the sight of the food during preparation was overwhelming? Did any single ingredient cause this reaction, either by sight or smell? Or was standing in a kitchen with residual smells part of the problem? Will a solid food really do? Would a drink be preferable? How does a thick liquid feel compared to a thin liquid? What taste and texture craving is the strongest when your sickness is at its peak? What taste and texture cravings emerge when you're feeling better?

In what room of your house or apartment do you most enjoy eating? Which room is the worst? Is there any correlation between the time of day and the place where you eat? There are several areas to explore in attempting to find a pattern in the bad times. Many small, invisible factors can help you feel better or, as most women prefer to say, "less worse." These factors all seem to revolve around the senses: smell, taste, motion, sight, hearing, touch, and stress. I've added motion and stress to the original quintet of senses because they seem to be highly significant factors in the successful management of morning sickness. Because they're difficult to measure, it's often hard for others to appreciate their intricate interrelationship, which contributes to morning sickness. Consideration of these aspects can make a difference in your sense of well-being.

My interviews with hundreds of pregnant women, from every socioeconomic level and cultural background, indicate that, although the problem of morning sickness is universal, the solutions are highly individual.

CRAVINGS

Back in 1957 two British researchers summarized information obtained from the BBC talk show *Is There a Doctor in the House?* on the topic of pregnancy. Women were asked to write in about their cravings. The reports from 820 pregnancies described 991 cravings, including 746 specific comments about food.

The most frequently craved foods were fruits (apples, oranges, lemons), followed by pickled food or raw cereal, then spices and condiments, and finally vegetables, especially tomatoes. About three-quarters of the women had two or more cravings simultaneously. One-quarter of the women found coffee and tea distasteful. The researchers were taken aback by the number of women who stressed the seriousness of their cravings and the lengths to which they went to satisfy them. The survey also noted that a small percentage of women craved nonfood items, such as coal, soap, laundry starch, clay, certain types of mud, disinfectant, and toothpaste. Apparently, the toothpaste used in Great Britain in the late 1950s was a powdered variety of which a main ingredient was baking soda (mainly sodium bicarbonate), an effective antacid.

Two-thirds of the pregnant women in another British study said they craved fruit because the juiciness satisfied their thirst. That study also found frequent cravings for strongly flavored foods, such as pickles, black (blood) pudding, licorice, potato crisps (chips), cheese, and kippers (smoked fish). Many women in the study said they found the sight of eggs revolting. Cravings for chocolates and other sweets were mentioned occasionally.

The craving for nonfood items is called pica. Although pica has been reported many times in the medical literature, the actual number of cases seems to be quite small. Pica can be extremely harmful to both the mother and the fetus, especially if the mother eats something as bizarre as inner tubes or air fresheners (which have each been reported only once).

If you have any unusual cravings, discuss them with a doctor or nutritionist, who can assess whether they're associated with any short-term or long-term nutritional or other problems. These strange urges may simply be an attempt to reduce debilitating nausea. A doctor may suggest a change in medication as well as prenatal vitamin supplements. A registered dietitian or nutritionist can provide additional food suggestions and perhaps recipes.

The range of foods eaten by women around the world during early pregnancy is highly variable, as the stories of the various women have revealed in this chapter.

YOUR ROAD TO SELF-IMPROVEMENT

Recording successful food choices and other variables is extremely helpful. Use the charts provided in this chapter. You can make as many copies of these charts as you need. The food lists that begin in the "Foods to Try" section are a good place to start. Make a check next to foods you've had success with. Cross out "no, never" foods and give "maybe" foods a question mark. It's important to evaluate familiar comfort foods. (Southern women often prefer bananas and mayonnaise on white bread, whereas several New England women told me their comfort food was cold seafood and spicy cocktail sauce—but it's different for everyone!) If your family's favorite comfort food has become repulsive to you, you need to let the rest of the family know—especially if your mother or another relative is coming to help out for a few days.

MORE PROBLEM SOLVING

Suppose you note that the worst time of the day is the morning. You can't even think about food or drink until 11 a.m. or your nausea rapidly escalates. But by 11 a.m., after adjusting to an upright position, making slow movements, and maintaining a quiet environment, you ask yourself what might ease your nausea, and *salty, dry,* and *crunchy* are the words that come to mind. How about potato chips? Do they appeal to you more than crackers? If so, there's no reason not to eat them. Other salty, dry foods might be cheese curls, popcorn, or pretzels.

Maybe ice cream works for you and sherbet doesn't. This is not the time to worry about the fat content. During a morning-sickness crisis, any type of calorie you can keep down is a successful calorie. In the field of clinical nutrition, we call this sick-day meal management.

Say the adjectives that come to mind are *wet/dry*, *crunchy*, and *cold*. Consider watermelon or a frozen fruit pop. If you think *tart*, *cold*, and *thick* may do the trick, try Italian lemon ice, lemonade mousse, or lemonade thickened with a modified corn starch supplement, called Thick-It or Thick 'n Easy.

Keep in mind that figuring out what you'll want to eat or drink 2 hours from now is like catching JELL-O in a fishnet— almost impossible. The invisible factors that control your condition (smells, hormones, blood chemistry, motion, fatigue, etc.) change constantly. I've worked with women whose taste buds screamed for salty foods when they felt the sickest. As they improved, they craved foods that were "sweet and earthy." Finding foods that work is like trying to hit a real moving target.

One woman reported that she couldn't get out of bed until she ate a pile of very salty crackers. At midmorning she drank lemonade and iced tea loaded with lemon. At noon she wanted oranges, and in mid-afternoon it was orange Creamsicles. If she didn't take an afternoon nap, nothing worked in the evening because her fatigue set off a bout of vomiting. After the nap, she got through the evening by eating chocolates. This woman—a nutrition-conscious college graduate—taught health, physical education, and aerobics.

She had struggled to resist urges to eat and drink lemonade, Creamsicles, and chocolates because she had considered them nonnutritious. Eating according to the guidelines her doctor's office gave at her second prenatal visit had met with no success. When she finally gave in to her cravings, she was able to function enough to care for her 2-year-old daughter and 5-year-old son. As the weeks went on, she was slowly able to add one or two of the recommended foods without precipitating an episode of vomiting.

Keep in mind that each food contains as many as 50 known nutrients. Add those factors to the widely varying textures and tastes of foods, and it's almost impossible to figure out why certain items work and others don't. But if you make a determined effort to record some of the general characteristics of the foods and beverages that work for you, you'll begin to see a pattern. It is okay to eat one food or one standard meal if that's the only thing you can keep down (this is *mono-eating*). Whatever works, use it.

DIET AND NAUSEA

A small study of 14 women who were in the first trimester of pregnancy suggested that a solid-food diet with a high protein content would more successfully alter the gastric dysrhythmias associated with the complaint of nausea than would diets of liquid or solid carbohydrates or fat. As with most studies on women with morning sickness, severe cases were excluded. These stomach wave patterns were monitored and recorded by a machine called an electrogastrogram. Again, these numbers are small, so it's important to listen to you own stomach. Jokingly, when I read this article, I told myself that when I did a re-write of my second book on morning sickness, titled *Take Two Crackers and Call Me in the Morning!* that I probably should change the title to *Take Two Pork Chops!*

FOODS TO TRY

The next few pages list the major food taste and texture categories. Keep in mind that you could probably add hundreds more to each list, and some foods can probably be cross-listed. Because tastes and attitudes about food and beverages are highly individual, there are no right or wrong answers. Trust your own experience and your gut.

When you look through these lists, you may wonder, where is balanced nutrition? If you're able to eat food from the four food groups regularly your morning sickness is probably very manageable, and that's great!

The compiled food lists help many women who are violently ill for long periods, who can't think of anything to make themselves better, and who need a fresh approach to finding foods and beverages they can keep down.

Consider those old stories that men tell of midnight drives to find pickles and ice cream and other strange food combinations. What could be more dissimilar? Analyze all the foods you crave and see what characteristics emerge. For example, pickles are low in calories; have a high water content; are high in salt, potassium, and fiber; and they have a distinct pungent aroma of vinegar, spices, and often garlic and dill. Ice cream is high in calories; is a solid liquid of sorts; is high in fat, low in salt, and low in potassium; and usually has a mild aroma, partly because it's cold. Nutritionally, pickles and ice cream are not the least bit similar, but each can serve a purpose.

Again, think back again to your overwhelming sick times and your choices of foods and beverages to prevent potentially serious dehydration. Ask your friends about their experiences. Remember, though, that once your morning-sickness crisis is over, eating a balanced diet is critical.

Grocery shopping can be an occasion for dread when you have morning sickness. You may be able to supply a list to the store and have an employee shop for you. (Some areas still have smaller stores that will accept telephone orders and deliver the groceries.) In some metropolitan areas, there are services, such as Peapod, that you might consider using. Peapod allows you to call and order your food, and they deliver it. Some of these services have a minimum order amount to get free delivery, and you might not get your food in the same day. That could be a problem. You also may not get exactly what you would have chosen for yourself, but that gamble may be well worth taking. If you have a family, others have to eat. Shopping for food and waiting in the checkout line is a big enough job when you are well. Consider saving yourself the time and aggravation by using services such as these when you are really feeling poorly.

The following lists of foods that many women find useful were compiled from my interviews over the past 15 years with women who had morning sickness. Your preferences for certain foods may change from time to time. It may be useful to write down the changes and date them; this information could show a trend when lots of variables come together. For example, when the weather changes from cold and brisk to hot and humid, in what direction do your food choices shift? Sharing your experiences with other women may unearth a lot of similarities.

When you have a choice between two products, I encourage you to buy organic or the least-processed ones available. It's also hard to know how much herbicide and pesticides are on fresh fruits and vegetables that come from overseas. Reportedly, there is more regulation in the United States on these items; however, given the amount of tainted meat we've read about in the news, how much inspection really goes on is a mystery to me.

Please note that I'm including brand names in these lists to help you find certain products. I have no stock in any of them.

Salty

Mashed potatoes with salt and parmesan cheese

Noodles with salt or grated cheese

Thin slices of ham (avoid deli products because of food safety; get it prepackaged and heat it then put back in the refrigerator until the meat reaches your desired temperature)

Thin slices of cheese

Grilled cheese sandwich

Grilled ham and cheese sandwich

Baked potato with cheese sauce and bacon bits

Ham and cheese rolled up with mustard

Tuna fish (limit to 3 servings a week because of mercury concerns)

Tomato juice

V-8 juice

Bloody Mary mix (without the alcohol)

Salted popcorn

Potato chips

Pretzels

Nacho chips

Macaroni and cheese

Quiche

Hotdog

Soydog

Relish

Ketchup

Cheeseburger

Vegetable soup

Tomato soup

String cheese

Cheese spread

Cooked baby pasta (pastina) with salt and parmesan cheese

Instant or regular grits with salt and cheddar cheese

Gatorade (it may not taste salty but it has a fair amount of sodium)

Sausage

Veggie breakfast patties

Bacon

Cup 'o Noodles

Cheese curls

Green apple (generally Granny Smith) sprinkled with salt

Anchovies

Caviar

Cheese and steak submarine sandwich

Deviled ham on crackers

Pickles (most of the time women grab dill pickles)

Cross out "no/never" items and add other favorite salty foods here.

_____

_____

Bitter/Tart/Sour

Pickles

English marmalade

Lemonade

Tamarinade

Extra-sour lemonade

Lemon mousse (see Chapter 12, "Recipes and Menus")

Whiskey sour mix (no alcohol) mixed with lemonade

Daiquiri mix (no alcohol) mixed with sparking water

Margarita mix (no alcohol)

Bloody Mary mix (no alcohol)

Grapefruit juice

Grapefruit juice with salt on the rim of the glass

Tom Collins mix (tonic, no alcohol)

Quinine (tonic) water

Tea (without milk or sugar)

Lemon wedges

Frozen lemon wedges

Frozen lime wedges

Frozen orange wedges

Fresh blueberries

Chinese plums

Tomato paste

Fresh cranberries

Sour apples

Concord grapes (jelly variety)

Lime juice sprinkled on apples

Limes

Rose's Lime juice (mixed with water)

Tamarinds

Sauerkraut

Salsa

Mustard (try different kinds)

Cheddar cheese with horseradish mixed in. The brand I tried and liked was Yaney's Fancy Horseradish Cheddar, which I found in the deli gourmet case at Star Market in Brighton, Massachusetts. (Try a grilled cheese sandwich with this for something different.)

Again, cross out "no/never" items and use the space below to write additional items.

_____

_____

EARTHY/YEASTY

Pesto (basically pine nuts, basil, and olive oil)

Brown rice

Mushrooms

Herbs such as thyme and marjoram

Mushroom soup

Sauteed mushrooms

Miso soup

Cream of potato soup

Pumpernickel bread

Black Russian rye bread

Bran cereal

Ground flaxseed meal

Wheat germ

Coarse-cut English or Irish oatmeal

Avocado

Spinach

Caesar salad (omit the raw egg in the dressing)

Baked potato

Mushroom pizza

Root beer

Cola

Brown cow (half milk and half cola)

Cheese bread

Ripe banana

Sourdough bread

Brie cheese (limit this because of the concern with soft cheeses and
    listeria; find a pasteurized brand or forget it)

Boursin cheese

Raisin toast

Lemon-flavored Portuguese sweet bread

Finnish coffee bread (with cardamom seeds)

Rusks (a form of dried biscuit)

Hot-and-sour soup

Rice pilaf

Hummus

Borscht

Tofu

Ricotta cheese

Yogurt cheese

Blue cheese (limit this because of the concern with soft cheeses and
    listeria; find a pasteurized brand or forget it)

Limburger cheese

Gouda cheese

Asparagus

Broccoli

Cauliflower

Brussels sprouts

Marinated mushrooms

Marinated artichokes

Bean burrito

Nuts

Smoked oysters

Clams (cooked and from inspected sources only)

Sardines

Mussels (cooked and from inspected sources only)

Pate (comes in several varieties, including pork liver, goose liver, salmon and vegetarian)

Homemade hot cocoa

Sunflower seeds

Nut butters (cashew, peanut)

Mugwort soba (Japanese buckwheat pasta with mugwort leaf)

Lox

Rooibos leaf tea, from Alvita, Twin Labs. I am familiar with Rooibos from traveling to Cape Town, South Africa, where it is called red bush tea. The tea has a very distinct flavor, and it's red, so it will stain your clothes if you aren't careful. It is used for stomach problems often, besides at the customary 4 p.m. tea and scones hour, which is wonderful! Rooibos rescued a colleague's problem with a screaming, colicy baby. All else had failed, so I gave my R.N. friend, Eileen, a bag of Rooibos from South Africa, and told her to make it up and put it in a baby bottle lukewarm. It worked.

A few weeks later, I ran into Eileen and she said the family had driven all over "The Cape" the weekend before, trying to find more Rooibos tea. "Where did you get it?" she asked. I told her she was driving around the wrong Cape—I found the tea in Cape Town, South Africa, not Cape Cod. Boy we had a great laugh over that one!

Pregnancy Tea, by Traditional Medicinals (contains raspberry, strawberry, and nettle leaves, spearmint, organic bitter fennel, organic rosehip, alfalfa leaf, and lemon verbena leaf).

Nut butters such as macadamia, almond, and cashew butter (by Maranantha)
Soy butter
Koku sesame rice cakes (by Lundberg)
Tamari seaweed rice cakes (by Lundberg)

Cross out the "no/never" items and add other favorite earthy/yeasty foods here.

_____

_____

CRUNCHY

Potato Crunchies (see Chapter 12)
Baked potato skins
Celery sticks
Diced celery, chopped walnuts, and whole cranberries in gelatin salad (see Walnut, Cranberry, and Celery Salad in Chapter 12)
Carrot sticks (to increase crunch, or water content, soak them in cold water for an 1 to 2 hours before eating)
Raw zucchini
Radishes
Lettuce
Crisp bacon
Fresh fruit cup

Fresh apple (red or green)

Cantaloupe

Honeydew melon

Fresh strawberries

Fresh blueberries

Pomegranates

Watermelon

Pears

Grapes

Potato chips

French fries

Cheese curls

Pretzels

Nuts

GORP (good old raisins and peanuts)

M&M's

Cucumbers

Pickles

Cherry tomatoes

Egg rolls

Sauerkraut on a hotdog

Corndog

Taco shells

Matzo crackers

Mergingue cookies (Trader Joe's has several flavors, including cinnamon and lemon)

Cross out the "no/never" items and add other favorite crunchy foods here.

_____

_____

BLAND

Mashed potatoes

Rice

Egg noodles

Custard

Vanilla pudding

Tapioca

Cream of wheat

Cream of rice

Oatmeal

White toast

Plain crackers

Vanilla wafers

Matzo crackers

Fortune cookies

Pancakes

Cottage cheese

Plain or vanilla yogurt

English muffins

Scones

Crumpets

Egg and plain bagels

Cross out the "no/never" items and add other favorite bland foods here.

_____

_____

Pre-preparing Bland Foods

Bland food is often thought of as the "white, yellow, and tan food group." Several foods in this group are staple items in our usual diet, such as potatoes, rice, and noodles. These days more people are buying prepackaged, prepared noodles, rice, and potatoes to save time. These tend to cost more and contain more salt and MSG and fewer nutrients. There is an economical, convenient, and nutritious alternative to prepackaged starches: cook ahead and freeze.

If you don't already have a microwave oven, now is a good time to consider buying a no-frills model. A toaster oven is also very useful for reheating food.

Mashed potatoes: Buy a 5-pound bag of nonbaking potatoes. If possible, have someone else peel and cook them all at once. Drain them and mash, adding the usual milk, trans-fat–free margarine or soy butter, and seasonings. Line small custard dishes or measuring cups with plastic, zippered sandwich bags. Scoop out 1/2 cup servings and place in bags. Squeeze all the air out and seal. Date each portion. Put all individual packages on a 9-by-12-inch cookie sheet to quick-freeze. When the packages are hard, put them all in one large plastic airtight freezer box or large plastic bag. Later, simply pull one out of the freezer, empty into a microwaveable custard dish, and heat in the microwave about one minute on high. For variety add grated cheese when reheating. Add some low-fat milk slowly, stir with a fork, and reheat, and you've got instant cream of potato soup. Frozen mashed potatoes last about 4 weeks in the freezer.

Noodles: Cook a 2-pound box of noodles. Drain and toss with olive or canola oil to prevent sticking. Fill zippered plastic bags with 1/2-cup servings, squeeze out the air, date, and freeze. Frozen noodles keep about 4 weeks in the freezer. To use, reheat as above.

Rice: Cook 2 pounds (or more) of rice according to package directions. Drain well. Divide into small freezer bags as directed above, squeeze out the air, date, and freeze. Frozen rice will keep well for 4 weeks in the freezer. Reheat as above.

If you want to make up a month's supply of basic cooked starch side dishes, do the potatoes, rice, and noodles in 1 day. Save pot-washing time by cooking the rice first. As the rice is cooling, add water to the empty pot to boil for the noodles. The small bit of rice starch left in the pot won't make a difference.

Cook the noodles according to the directions on the package while dividing the cooked and cooled rice for the freezer. Once the rice strainer is empty, the noodles are probably ready to rinse and drain. After draining, put the noodles back into the large pot and toss them with a bit of margarine to prevent sticking. Empty the noodles back into the strainer to cool. Then proceed with the packaging. Add more water to the cooking pot to cook the potatoes. Once the potatoes are cooked and drained, mash them in the same pot.

One cautionary note: There are smells attached to cooking even these bland foods. The boiling water and vapors carry small amounts of starch molecules, which have distinctive aromas. Even these mildest of aromas can trigger an episode of nausea. Be sure any cooking is done with opened windows and the exhaust fan on high speed. It would be preferable to give these few pages to a good friend or family member to execute rather than you.

Hot cereal: Making a large batch of hot cereal at one time saves both time and money. Use the conventional oatmeal or hot cereal of your choice. Make 6 servings. After it cools, refrigerate it. To use, simply scoop out a single serving into a bowl, cover with a ceramic saucer and microwave. Around mid-afternoon, you can add a scoop of cold cereal to a coffee mug, add milk, and put in microwave for 1 to 2 minutes for a hot, satisfying, quick pick-me-up, semi-drink. Individual portions of oatmeal can also be successfully frozen in individual containers. Thaw and reheat in the microwave.

By the way, *never* microwave food in plastic products! The chemicals in the containers come out with heating and there are concerns of increased health risks.

Cream of wheat: I made this up using cranberry juice instead of water, which gave it a little zap!

Make hot cereals using milk instead of water to get in more calcium. Or use half milk and half water if you can't do much milk because of lactose intolerance.

SOFT

French toast (syrup optional)
Mashed potatoes
Rice
Noodles
Ice cream
Custard
Canned peaches and pears
Grilled cheese sandwich
Tortellini
Stuffed baked potatoes
Cream of wheat
Cream of rice
Pancakes
Yogurt
Cottage cheese
Canned fruit
Angel-food cake
Pound cake

Pudding

Danish pastry

Cross out the "no/never" items and add other favorite soft foods here.

_____

_____

SWEET

Candy

Cake

Canned fruit

Ice cream

Sherbet

Dried fruit

Sugared cereal

Jam

Jelly

Syrup

Flavored instant hot cereal

Cross out the "no/never" items and add other favorite sweet foods here.

_____

_____

FRUITY

Fresh fruit

Fruit in cereal

Jam on toast

Grilled ham and pineapple sandwich

Peanut butter and jelly sandwich

Canned fruit

Popsicle

Fruit leather

Dried fruit

Fruit blintz

Fruit compote

Cross out "no/never" items and add other favorite fruity foods here.

_____

_____

WET

Seltzer

Tonic

Milk

Milkshake

Juice

Juicy fresh fruit

Slush

Pureed fruit

Water (see the note that follows)

Thick and cold liquids

Most women complain that their tap water has a funny taste or smell. Sometimes that is caused by algae that grow in the summer in the local reservoir or by sulfur or chlorine. It might also be caused by metals that leak from old pipes or plastic components from newer synthetic pipes. Women in a queasy crisis often have more success with flavored bottled waters.

Cross out "no/never" items and add other favorite wet foods here.

_____

_____

DRY

Crackers

Bread

Toast

Cookies

Cereal

Dried fruit

Beef jerky

Dried beef

Thai tea (see the note that follows)

Freeze-dried ice cream (available in large science museums, at sporting goods/camping supply stores, or from the National Air and Space Museum in Washington, D.C.)

Not many liquids produce a "dry" sensation, but Thai tea seems to be one of them. If you don't have Thai tea but want to try something similar, simply add 1 teaspoon of vanilla to a cup of hot regular tea.

Cross out "no/never" items and add other favorite dry foods here.

_____

_____

SPICY

Ginger ale

Homemade ginger ale (see Chapter 12 for the recipe)

Gingerbread

Gingerbread cookies

Salsa

Chili peppers

Hot dipping sauce

Tabasco sauce

Seafood cocktail sauce

Guacamole

Curry

Cinnamon toast

Spices of any kind

Marinades of all sorts to flavor your protein source: chicken, fish, other meats, and tofu. (I've been experimenting with ones that have ginger as an ingredient: Trader Joe's Black Bean and Ginger gives chicken a real kick! Wasabi Teriyaki is another sauce with zap.)

Cross out "no/never" items and add other favorite spicy foods here.

_____

_____

HARD

Hard candy

Rusks

Biscotti

Crackers

Toasted bagel

Popsicles

Fresh fruit (apple, pear, peach)

Dried fruit

Nuts

Beef jerky

Frozen chocolate chips

Frozen jelly beans

Ice chips

Frozen fruit-juice ice chips

Meringue cookies

Cracker Jacks

Cross out "no/never" items and add other favorite hard foods here.

_____

_____

Hot

Just-cooked foods

Foods heated in a microwave

Hot liquids (if you drink tea, you may have more success if it's tea
   piping hot rather than lukewarm)

Baked fruit

Freshly baked custard or pudding

Instant hot cereal

Spicy foods

Soups

Hot chocolate

Hot milk with a teaspoon of honey

Cross out "no/never" items and add other favorite hot items here.

_____

_____

COLD

Frozen desserts

Yogurt

Ice cream

Sherbet

Frozen fruit pops

Leftover chicken legs

Potato salad

Tortellini salad

Fruit soup

Iced tea

Whole-wheat pasta salad with celery and salmon mixed in with a
  little mayo

Iced herbal tea (in moderation due to unresolved controversy about
  the exact ingredients in many teas)

Lassi (Indian salty yogurt drink; see Chapter 12 for the recipe)

Milkshake

Fruit shake

Chocolate milk

Strawberry-flavored milk

Leftover refrigerated pizza

Mousse

Frozen grapes

Pickles

Cross out "no/never" items and add other favorite cold foods and beverages here.

_____

_____

PUNGENT/AROMATIC

Hot mustard sauce

Ginger

Wasabi coated chick peas

Ginseng tea (in moderation)

Mint tea (hot or cold)

Licorice

Anise

Rosemary

Garlic

Dill

Cinnamon

Other herbs and spices

Zesty tomato chips (by Terra Chips)

Baked spicy black bean dip (by Guiltless Gourmet, online at http://www.guiltlessgourmet.com)

Cross out "no/never" items and add other favorite pungent/aromatic foods and beverages here.

_____

_____

LEMON

Lemon crème pudding mix, by Morinaga Nutritional Foods, Inc. from Torrance, California. This is 100 percent vegan, you make it with tofu and water.

Lemon Snaps, by Mi-del, part of American Natural Specialty Brands from Augustine, Florida. They also have gluten-free cookies in chocolate, pecan, and arrowroot flavors.

Lemon meringue cookies by Trader Joe's.

Celestrial Seasonings has three beverage flavors, packed in four 11-ounce ready-to-go containers: kiwi-lemon, lemon-zinger black tea, and ginger lemon green tea. Get more information online at http://www.celestialseasonings.com.

GINGER

Pumpkin-ginger cookies, by Immaculate Baking Co. in Flat Rock, North Carolina. (Call (888) 32MOJOS for more information.

Spiced taro chips. by Terra Chips, are a potato chip alternative that contains ginger and lemon. Call (800) 434-4246 for more information or go to http://www.terrachips.com.

Black Bean and Ginger Sauce from Trader Joe's. I was very pleasantly surprised with the outcome of marinating a small swordfish steak in this product. First, I sautéed three huge carrots cut diagonally in a small amount of olive oil for 3 minutes, until they looked toasty, I put in the 3-ounce marinated swordfish cut into 1-inch cubes, put on a pot lid, and turned down the heat. Brown rice was cooking quietly on a burner and broccoli steaming quickly in the microwave. Within 5 minutes, dinner was ready to go. The label on the sauce jar says "great with fish and chicken," but it gave no recipes for cooking with either. I would venture a guess that tofu marinated overnight and sautéed with a combo of carrots, one clove of garlic, and a few onions would be tasty. But maybe not for the queasy woman.

GLUTEN-FREE FOODS

All-Natural Frookies are sweetened with fruit juice and are wheat-
and gluten-free. They come in chocolate, vanilla, and peanut
butter flavors. Call (888) FROOKIE to order.

Brown Rice Chips by Eden Foods. Get more information or order
online at http://www.edenfoods.com.

Original Rice Bran Crackers, by Healthy Valley, are wheat- and
gluten-free. Call (800) 423-4846 to order.

Wild Rice Cakes, by Lundberg.

SICK-DAY MEAL PLANS

A few sick-day meal plans that utilize the previous lists are provided
here as examples only. I don't insist that you eat exactly in this
fashion, particularly if you can tolerate other, more nutritious foods.
A daily guide to more healthful eating can serve as a goal when your
crisis is under control. Also note that food tastes are purely
subjective. Feel free to re-categorize each food into your own
compartments.

SICK-DAY MEAL PLAN (SALTY)

7 a.m. (or first meal of the day) 8 salted soda crackers, matzos, or
pretzels.

8 a.m. 6 potato chips.

9 a.m. 1/2 cup Gatorade.

10 a.m. 1/2 sliced green apple, sprinkled with coarse salt.

11 a.m. 4 or 5 cheese curls or 1 stick beef jerky.

Noon. 1/2 cup cooked pasta with 1 tablespoon grated parmesan cheese.

1 p.m. 1/2 cup Gatorade or nonalcoholic Bloody Mary mix.

2 p.m. 6 to 8 potato chips.

3 p.m. 1/2 cup mashed potatoes with grated cheese.

4 p.m. 1/2 cup chicken noodle soup.

5 p.m. 1/2- or 1-ounce thinly sliced American cheese on a salted rice cake.

6 p.m. 4 or 5 thinly sliced cucumbers, marinated in white vinegar and salt. Eat the thoroughly washed skins if possible for the fiber; or try a few pickles.

7 p.m. 1/2 cup cooked pastina with salt added. Cook the pastina in half water and half milk to add a bit more nutrition.

8 p.m. 1 ounce thinly sliced ham with 1 or 2 diced cherry tomatoes rolled up inside.

Continue munching until bedtime.

SICK-DAY MEAL PLAN (TART/BITTER/SOUR)

7 a.m. (or first meal of the day) rinse your mouth out with ice-cold water with lemon slices in it or try 1 or 2 lemon sour balls.

8 a.m. 1/4 cup lemon pie filling with extra lemon rind or juice added.

9 a.m. 1/2 cup lime juice mixed with 1/4 cup seltzer.

10 a.m. 1/2 pomegranate.

11 a.m. 1/2 cup (nonalcoholic) whiskey sour mix.

Noon. 1/2 cup frozen grapes rolled in lime and sugar.

1 p.m. 1/2 cup tonic water with a grapefruit slice in it

2 p.m. 1-2 tablespoons seafood cocktail sauce with lemon wedges and 1 or 2 (or more) freshly cooked shrimp.

3 p.m. 1/2 cup homemade lemonade or Tamarinade.

4 p.m. 1/4 turkey sandwich on a whole-wheat roll with tangy mustard.

5 p.m. 1/2 cup lime pudding (adjust with extra lime juice) or a piece of key lime pie.

6 p.m. 1/2 cup homemade cranberry juice.

7 p.m. 1 or 2 gingersnaps with low-fat ricotta or cottage cheese on top, sprinkled with nutmeg or ginger.

8 p.m. Repeat any of these as desired.

Continue munching until bedtime.

SICK-DAY MEAL PLAN (BLAND)

7 a.m. (or first meal of the day) 4 unsalted oyster crackers.

8 a.m. 1/2 egg matzo cracker.

9 a.m. 1/2 cup instant cream of wheat or grits with milk.

10 a.m. 1/2 ripe banana blended with 1/2 cup milk to make a milkshake.

11 a.m. 1/4 cup applesauce.

Noon. 1/2 cup quick pineapple yogurt blender pudding, or substitute canned pears for pineapple.

1 p.m. 1/2 cup apricot nectar.

2 p.m. 1/2 cup instant hot rice.

3 p.m. 1/2 cup homemade tapioca or rice pudding.

4 p.m. 1/2 cup fine-curd cottage cheese with 1/4 cup diced guava added.

5 p.m. 1/2 cup cream of potato soup, hot or cold.

6 p.m. 1-inch square of Noodle Kugel (see Chapter 12 for this recipe).

7 p.m. 3 animal crackers and 1/2 cup warm milk. Add vanilla to milk for a change.

8 p.m. 2 tablespoons whipped ricotta cheese on 1/2 cup warmed applesauce.

Continue munching until bedtime.

SICK-DAY MEAL PLAN (CRUNCHY)

7 a.m. (or first meal of the day) 3 melba toasts or 1 rice cake.

8 a.m. 1/2 cup freshly sliced apple and 1/2 ounce cheddar cheese.

9 a.m. 1/2 cup watermelon cubes or shrimp chips. These are generally imported from Vietnam—made from shrimp, tapioca starch and egg white. Although you can make them, it's easier to call a Vietnamese restaurant and see if you can buy some, or look for them at an Oriental grocery store.

10 a.m. 1/2 cup wheat and fruit cereal with 1/4 cup milk.

11 a.m. 2 oatmeal raisin nut cookies.

Noon. 1/2 cup frozen grapes or gingered grapefruit (sugar and ground ginger sprinkled over fresh grapefruit).

1 p.m. 1/2 cup gazpacho, hot or cold.

2 p.m. 1 cucumber and watercress sandwich (use very thin bread).

3 p.m. 1/4 cup GORP or 1/4 cup homemade granola with 1/4 cup milk.

4 p.m. 3 or 4 mandarin orange slices with slivered almonds and a leaf of Boston or Bibb lettuce.

5 p.m. 1/2 bacon, lettuce, and tomato sandwich on toast.

6 p.m. 1/2 cup Waldorf Salad (see Chapter 12 for the recipe) with 1/4 cup cottage cheese mixed in.

7 p.m. 1/2 cup mild (homemade) chicken broth with 1/4 cup chopped bok choy and 1/2 cup julienned carrots, cooked al dente, and added.

8 p.m. 1 or 2 cheese crunchy "crackers." Here's the recipe: On a nonstick baking sheet lay out several 1-by-1-by-1/4–inch slices of cheddar cheese and bake in oven until melted and slightly browned. When the cheese melts and browns slightly, remove it

from the oven. When cool, store the cheese in a jar in the refrigerator. Eat within 3 days.

Continue munching until bedtime.

SICK-DAY MEAL PLAN (SWEET)

7 a.m. (or first meal of the day) 2 shortbread or sugar cookies.

8 a.m. 1-inch square Noodle Kugel (see Chapter 12).

9 a.m. 1/2 cup grape juice.

10 a.m. 1 slice raisin toast with cinnamon sugar on top.

11 a.m. 1/2 cup cherry mousse.

Noon. 1 or 2 yogurt-cottage cheese pancakes, topped with Lyle's Golden Syrup or maple syrup.

1 p.m. 1/2 cup cherry Gatorade or chocolate milk.

2 p.m. 1/4 to 1/2 cup raspberry or orange sherbet.

3 p.m. 1/2 cup thawed frozen strawberries with juice over a ladyfinger

with whipped cream.

4 p.m. 1 small slice Easy Refrigerator Pie (see Chapter 12 for the recipe).

5 p.m. 1/2 cup peach milkshake (3 peach halves blended with 1/4 cup milk).

6 p.m. 1/2 cup baked flan (see Chapter 12 for the recipe).

7 p.m. 1/2 cup cranberry (sweetened) or apricot juice.

8 p.m. 1 or 2 pieces of dried fruit.

Continue munching until bedtime.

SICK-DAY MEAL PLAN (EARTHY)

7 a.m. (or first meal of the day) 1 whole-grain rice cake.

8 a.m. 1/2 cup muesli and 1/4 cup plain soy milk.

9 a.m. 4 or 5 macadamia nuts.

10 a.m. 1/2 Portuguese pancake with lemon curd.

11 a.m. 1/2 cup Ginger Sundae (see Chapter 12 for the recipe).

Noon. Sautéed mushrooms over wheat toast.

1 p.m. 1/4 avocado or a handful of shrimp chips.

2 p.m. 1/4 cup prune juice or a slice of Flowerpot Bread (see Chapter 12 for the recipe).

3 p.m. 1 piece Pumpkin-Cheese Pie (see the recipe in Chapter 12) or 1/2 cup pumpkin custard.

4 p.m. 1 2-inch piece Rice-Carrot Casserole (cold or hot) cut in thin slices (see Chapter 12 for the recipe).

5 p.m. 1/2 cup Lemon and Brown Rice Chicken Casserole (see Chapter 12 for the recipe).

6 p.m. 1/2 cup Orange Pudding and Hot Nutmeg and Ginger Milk, Digestive Tea, or Barley Tea (see Chapter 12 for the recipes).

7 p.m. 1 tbsp vegetable pate or liverwurst on rye crackers.

8 p.m. 1 or 2 sardines on 1/2 slice oatmeal toast.

Continue munching until bedtime.

ADDING VARIETY TO YOUR EATING HABITS

To add some interesting variety, see how your taste buds like eating upside down. What I mean by this is if you usually assemble your sandwich in with bread, mustard, ham, cheese, butter, and bread in that order of layers, turn it upside down and eat it. The flavors will hit your mouth in different places. Or add extra flavors between each layer such as bread, mustard, ham, mustard, cheese, mustard, and bread. Try adding a small layer of jam to a cheese sandwich. A friend of mine from overseas acquainted me with this trick.

Your taste buds will most likely cry out for a variety of flavors throughout the day, and you'll mix and match foods from all of the food lists. When you make a chart, you'll probably find that particular foods and beverages will predominate at the nadir and zenith your nausea cycle. What's important is to find foods that work. I map or chart them according to where they fall in that cycle. After a cycle or two, this recorded information will most likely show a pattern and help you predict which foods may work for you.

ETHNIC AND CULTURAL OFFERINGS

I scanned all the cookbooks I own and relegated recipes to various categories. This is only my opinion and assessment, so it's not definitive! Please do consider foods from other regions. You may not be able to make a recipe yourself, but your friends could. Or there is always take-out food from restaurants.

SALTY

Spinach with anchovies (Espinacas con Anchoas, from Venzuela). This dish has only four ingredients: spinach or Swiss chard, olive oil, anchovies, and freshly ground pepper.

Salted cod with eggs (Pudim de Bacalhau com Ovos from Brazil). This is a traditional breakfast food including salt cod, capers, tomatoes, onions eggs and cheese.

SOUR

Avgolemono soup (from Greece). This is chicken broth with whole eggs or egg yolks mixed in with lemon juice and corn starch. It has a nice zing.

Baked potatoes oregano (Patates sto fourno rigantes from Greece). This is a casserole of grated potatoes mixed with olive oil and juice of one lemon, with a pinch of oregano and salt and pepper added, and baked.

Hot and sour fish soup (Sayur Asam Ikan from Java). Besides having fish in this, it is seasoned with tamarind and hot chilies.

BITTER/TART

Winter's seasonal salad (Salata na Sezon Simowy from Poland). This dish includes spinach, lettuce, onion slices, and radishes.

Cabbage, leek, and orange salad (Salata z Kapusty, Porow i Pomarañczy from Poland). This contains oranges, mixed with shredded red cabbage, lemon juice, chopped leek, honey, and olive oil

Spinach and lemon soup (from the Cooperhill House in Ireland). This soup is made with fresh spinach in chicken broth and grated zest and juice of a lemon.

Orange or lemon rolls (Pomeranzenbrötchen from Germany).

SWEET

Banana sweet soup (Che Chuoi from Vietnam).

Bean curd dessert (Dau Hu from Vietnam). This one looks like a high-protein item.

Pork chops with dried fruit (Chuletas de Cerdo con Frutas from the Dominican Republic). Change the flavor of meats by adding a variety of dried fruits. In this case, you add prunes (now called dried plums), dried apricots, and dried pears.

CRUNCHY

Carrot salad (Carot ngam dam from Vietnam). This salad is made with vinegar and sugar.

White radish (Cu cai from Vietnam).

Pistachio canape (Kanape me Fistiki from Greece). This contains softened cream cheese on bread rounds, sprinkled with pistachio nuts. You can use walnuts, too.

Almond cookie (Ergolavi from Greece). The recipe calls for 6 cups of almonds to 3 cups of sugar and 3 egg whites. These cookies have no fat and are high in protein. I'm sure you might be able to decrease the amount of sugar a bit, but probably not by more than 1/2 cup. Recipes are a balance of ingredients to hold things together.

Horseradish with apples (Jablecny Kren from former Czechoslovakia). This is a raw, salad-type item with some lemon juice in it, and it is generally served with meat. It has a bit of a kick.

FRUITY

Candied orange or lemon peel (Kandovani Pomerancover a critronove kury from former Czechoslovakia). This is an elegantly simple recipe for making your own candied citrus rind. Although it has a high percentage of sugar, a bit here or there at work might be just the thing to keep your stomach under control.

WET

Cucumber and grapefruit salad (Tha Khwa Thee Shauk Thee Thoke from Burma). Ingredients besides cucumber and grapefruit are little bit of onion, fish sauce, chili peppers, and spinach.

Sorrel (from Jamaica). To make this beverage, start with dried sorrel and add cloves, orange peel, grated fresh ginger, water, sugar and a small amount of white rice. Season the mixture with nutmeg. The original recipe calls for a tweak of rum or brandy, but forget that!

Lemonade (Lemouroudji from West Africa). This beverage combines freshly grated ginger root, a dash of cayenne pepper, water, sugar, and juice from 1 pound of lemons. The cayenne is optional.

Hohoise ice (Indian tea ice). This is a medicinal tea from Arizona. Hohoise can be mail-ordered. Besides Hohoise leaves, this tea contains anise and cinnamon.

DRY

Honey almond cookies (Pierniczki z Migdalami from Poland). Besides honey, eggs, flour, almonds, the spices included in these cookies are ginger, nutmeg, and cinnamon.

TART

Onion salad (Cibulovy Salat from former Czechoslovakia). Onions should be cooked in a water-vinegar mixture.

Kohlrabi salad (Brukvovy Salat from former Czechoslovakia). Young kohlrabi are used and tossed with a vingarette or mayonnaise dressing. This salad is both tart and crunchy.

Tart lemon custard (from The Rosleague Manor in Ireland). The four ingredients are heavy cream, eggs, sugar, and lemon juice. This is a baked dish.

HOT

Steamed rice pudding (Ryzovy Pudnik from former Czechoslovakia). This nutritious-looking recipe includes ground almonds and eggs, so it has some good-quality protein.

Hot peppers in milk (Ajies en leche from Venezuela). This is an interesting sauce, served with poultry, fish, or other meat. An optional ingredient is mint leaves.

Maple Ginger Tea (from a Native American recipe). The secret ingredient is a dash of paprika.

Cardamom and Coriander rice (Kotmir Illaichi-Wale Chaaval from India). The secret ingredients in here are cardamom pods, a little cayenne pepper, and freshly chopped coriander or parsley.

COLD

Fruit soup (Fruktsuppe from Norway). This soup contains prunes, raisins, dried apricots, unsweetened cherries, and juice cooked with a cinnamon stick, a little sugar, and tapioca. It is served cold.

Watermelon ice delight (Tarbooi ki Kheer from India), Essentially, this is watermelon ice cream.

BLAND

Paraguayan corn bread (Sopa Paraguaya from Paraguay). This interesting recipe has two types of cheese added—cottage cheese and cheddar cheese—besides eggs and milk. This is a good source of protein and calcium.

Potato soup (Potetsuppe from Norway). This is a simple recipe with a little parsley tossed in at the end. It is made with milk, so it is a good way to get in your calcium.

Oatmeal soup (Haferflockensuppe from Germany). This isn't your ordinary oatmeal; two egg yolks are beaten and added to the oatmeal. Cream is also an ingredient. It would probably work fine to substitute evaporated milk for the cream.

SMOOTH

Avocado salad (Ensalada de Aguacate from Columbia). This contains four simple ingredients: ripe avocado, white-wine vinegar, salt, and freshly ground black pepper.

Pineapple custard (Flan de Pina from Columbia). The simple ingredients in this recipe include unsweetened pineapple juice, sugar, and eggs.

Pumpkin Corn soup with ginger lime cream. This bland soup from Native Americans of the Southwest adds a zest with a garnish of ginger lime cream.

MUSHY

Rice porridge (Risengrynsgrot from Norway). This is a traditional breakfast item: white rice cooked in milk with a little butter and salt. It is generally served hot with a little cinnamon and sugar on top and additional milk if preferred.

Glutinous rice and mango (Khao Niew-Mamoung from Thailand). The rice is soaked overnight and mixed with coconut milk, sugar, and 1 or 2 ripe mangos.

SPICY

Ginger roast beef (Hovezi Pecene Na Zazvoru from former Czechoslovakia). This is a traditional dish. The roast beef is dusted with powdered ginger before it is roasted.

Spiced string beans (Sambal Goreng Buntjies from Java). Ingredients in this dish include string beans, coconut milk, shrimp, salam leaves, and tamarind seasoning.

Spiced eggs (Telor Bumbu Bali from Bali). Hard-cooked eggs are seasoned with onions, dried red hot chili peppers, soy sauce, ginger, and tamarind.

Spicy coconut milk soup (Laksa Lemak from Malaysia). This is an elaborate soup with many ingredients, including macadamia nuts.

EARTHY

Cauliflower with straw mushrooms (Bong Cai Xao Nam Romz from Vietnam).

Smoked herring spread (Pomazanka Z Uzenacu from former Czechoslavakia). This spread is an interesting combination of grated Swiss cheese, mashed sardines (high omega-3 food), a bit of grated onion, butter (substitute Garden Soy), and paprika.

Brown soda bread (from the Park Hotel Kenmare, Ireland). This bread uses wheat germ and whole-wheat flour, so it doesn't require the extra time for rising.

Lemon lentils (Nimbu Masoor Dal from India). Cinnamon, ginger, and lemon juice are among the list of ingredients.

FIZZY

Ginger beer (from Jamaica). This beverage starts with 1/2 pound of freshly peeled ginger. Added to it are lime juice, sugar, and active dry yeast. It takes 2 weeks to make.

Chapter 10

Complications of Severe and/or Extended Morning Sickness

DAVID

"Does lightning ever strike twice in the same spot?" David asked. Having endured morning sickness secondhand with his wife's first pregnancy, he thought it couldn't happen again. Among the issues he tried to deal with was a continuing feeling of helplessness. During her bouts of severe vomiting, Laura was unable to look after their 2-year-old son, Leif. Laura would put him into his crib to keep him safe and call David, begging him to come home to help her get Leif ready for bed because she could not manage by herself. He was often able to calm her down over the phone and say that nothing bad would happen if the baby slept in clothes and not pajamas.

David found concentrating at work difficult because he knew things were probably in shambles at home. Three times during the second pregnancy Laura was hospitalized, leaving Leif with David's parents. Laura, having lost 10 pounds by week 10, was reported to be malnourished. He had overheard this news one evening when he came to visit, which was during change of shift for the nursing staff. The nurses were in the back room, off to the side of the unit desk, and he needed to wait to register while the secretary was on the phone with a doctor. He was horrified! Malnutrition? He had done his best to try to feed and care for her—hearing that word floored him beyond belief. He loved his wife dearly and certainly would never have neglected her for all the tea in China! He worried about what the doctors would be thinking of him. "After this pregnancy is over, that's it!" David announced once he kissed his pale wife hello. Both of them agreed that the difficulties involved in having children were just overwhelming, and they decided on permanent birth control once Babe Numero Dos arrived. He vowed to scheduled himself for a vasectomy once Laura was home postpartum and able to function by herself.

David happened to run into the registered dietitian he suspected was responsible for this malnutrition label—me. As a member of the Obstetrician High-Risk Team, I covered all the patients, even though Laura and David were cared for by a private obstetrician group. Morning sickness affects even those living in high socioeconomic zip codes. I explained to David, that the fact that Laura lost weight and hadn't eaten well in weeks was no reflection on his love and devotion. Although at this point in time there are no specific criteria for malnutrition for the pregnant woman, there have been standards for hospitalized patients in general. We tweak those standards for pregnant women who don't eat, because advocating for the unborn baby is *very* important.

CRITERIA FOR MALNUTRITION

Malnutrition is not just a third-world problem, although that's what most people think. In fact, in major teaching hospitals, about 50 percent of folks admitted, outside of the obstetrical population, are at risk for or have frank malnutrition.

A few years ago, our nutrition department did a patient survey as part of a project during National Nutrition Month: We counted up all our patients with malnutrition or risk factors for malnutrition in 2 days. As part of a contest, we asked all hospital staff to guess the average percentage of patients who were at risk for malnutrition. (We gave out two prizes for the closest answers). We encouraged every employee to enter. Guesses were all over the place, and we published our results internally as well as in professional literature. The answer, excluding the obstetrical population, was about 52 percent— meaning every other patient!

There are institutionally created standards to classify patients with malnutrition. In our hospital, not eating for 1 week gives you one point. Loosing 10 pounds in 2 weeks gives you another point. Because our hospital is a tertiary care center, by the time patients are admitted, they have spent a lot of time in other hospitals or sick at home, not eating well. Our threshold for the diagnosis of malnutrition may be different from other hospitals because all of our registered dietitians were asked about their opinions based on the populations they cared for. In some cases we use three of six criteria for classifying a patient with some degree of malnutrition. We also created a category termed "nonspecific protein calorie malnutrition," where clinical judgment is allowed some weight when the clinical suspicion is high for poor nutrition.

Just for a ballpark idea of how malnutrition is classified, Table 10.1 gives some parameters for overall malnutrition, based on the International Classification of Diseases, ninth edition, clinical modification (ICD-9-CM).

Table 10.1 International Classification of Disease Parameters for Malnutrition.

ICD-9-CM	Diagnosis/Description	Criteria/Characteristics
260.0	Kwashiorkor	At least 90 percent of weight for height
		Serum albumin less than 3.0 mg/dL
		Edema (fluid collection), muscle loss
		Neurological changes, loss of vigor
261.0	Marasmus, severe chronic calorie deficiency	Usual weight less than 80 percent normal
		Weight loss over 10 percent in 6 months with muscle wasting or loss
		Chronically deficit energy intake
		Lethargy, lack of vigor
		Serum albumin over 3.0 mg/dL
262.0	Other protein energy malnutrition	Less than 60 percent weight for height
		Serum albumin less than 3.0
		High risk for infection, poor wound healing
263.0	Malnutrition of moderate degree	60–75 percent of usual body weight
		Serum albumin 3.0–3.5 mg/dL
263.1	Malnutrition of mild degree	75–90 percent of standard weight for height
		Serum albumin 3.5–5.0 mg/dL

(Kwashiorkor and marasmus are African words for starvation. Simply said, Kwashiorkor is skin and bones with a bloated potbelly, and maramus is skin and bones.)

Although there is no special category for malnutrition in pregnancy, I add to the weight loss the lack of weight gain expected in pregnancy. In Laura's case, she had a net weight loss of 10 pounds.

But by 10 weeks, she should have gained 3 to 5 pounds, so her gross weight loss—in my opinion—was 13 to 15 pounds. The acceptable range for the serum protein albumin in pregnancy drops to 2.5 to 4.5 because of normal fluid changes. Using serum albumin as a factor in the current malnutrition criteria isn't very useful in pregnancy. Albumin levels are falsely high with dehydration. Obtaining vitamin and mineral laboratories to assess for malnutrition is sometimes helpful, but these studies are expensive and take time to come back. Unfortunately, there isn't a good set of normal vitamin and mineral charts based on trimester of pregnancy. With 4,000,000 babies born in the United States every year, you'd think this would be available!

Laura's situation of not eating well for weeks and losing 10 pounds gave her a secondary diagnosis of nonspecific protein calorie malnutrition along with her admitting diagnosis of hyperemesis gravidarum at 10 weeks. I showed David the guidelines we used and said that her nutritional progress would be monitored closely. If we didn't see improvement with her eating a multiple small meals every day and receiving fluid support with intravenous vitamins, we'd need to consider more aggressive nutritional interventions to ensure a healthy mother and healthy pregnancy. David was reassured with this information.

DOES MORNING SICKNESS MEAN SOMETHING IS WRONG?

You and your family will want to know that plain, garden-variety morning sickness is not a sign that something is wrong with the pregnancy. In fact, statistics indicate that women who experience nausea, in particular, are more likely to have successful pregnancies than those who do not. Morning sickness has also been associated with fewer spontaneous abortions and early miscarriage.

In 1972 the National Institute of Neurological Diseases and Stroke investigated the effects of morning sickness, looking for the likelihood of an adverse outcome. Finding nothing significant, they cautiously concluded that there did not appear to be any greater risk of delivering a low-birth-weight baby nor any increased risk of deformity or congenital malformation because of nausea and vomiting. We are talking morning sickness here, though, and not frank hyperemesis gravidarum.

Most women who are affected by nausea, vomiting, and weight loss worry about the well-being of their babies. A woman may wonder, "how can a baby grow if I'm not eating? Isn't the baby affected by my weight loss?"

A German research team seems to have come up with an explanation of why babies born to mothers with morning sickness aren't noticeably smaller. For some reason yet undetermined, the researchers found that the blood flow to the uterus of women hospitalized with hyperemesis gravidarum was at least twice that of a healthy pregnant woman. Maybe this finding suggests that there is a compensatory system that helps protect the fetus from the mother's inability to consume adequate nutrition. This was just one study and has not been repeated, so the information has limited utility. In addition, although we have limited details, we aren't sure whether the women were on intravenous fluids or not.

If you are not getting supervised prenatal care, you could be at risk for serious dehydration and electrolyte imbalance. Adverse outcomes resulting from untreated vomiting in pregnancy may be more common in societies where medical care is not readily accessible and medical reporting is rare. For instance, when I cared for one woman who was hospitalized with severe morning sickness, her boyfriend told me about a distant cousin who died in a remote village in Nigeria because of untreated vomiting several years earlier. After I heard this story, I tried to obtain international statistics about hyperemesis gravidarum, but was unsuccessful.

Refractory vomiting, or vomiting that does not subside with a full complement of standard medical attention, may be a sign of other significant medical problems that are beyond the scope of this book: diseases of the gallbladder, kidney, liver, pancreas, appendix, intestinal tract, and thyroid, to name but a few.

For many women the nausea and vomiting of morning sickness are occasional, not continual, and are limited to the first trimester of pregnancy. However, women with severe and extended morning sickness are at risk for other problems besides poor nutrition:

Inadequate weight gain

Marginal fluid consumption

Constipation

Anemia

Tooth and gum problems

Irritation of the throat and nose

Early satiety and overeating

Muscle loss from prolonged bed rest

Heightened physical discomfort

Sleep deprivation

The impact of each of these can be minimized with increased awareness of the potential problems and by making better food choices when possible. Each of these factors, although related to your overall diet, is important for special reasons.

INADEQUATE WEIGHT GAIN

Women don't all need to gain the same amount of weight during pregnancy. The charts in the appendix provide a suggested rate of gain, which depends on your prepregnancy weight. An underweight woman needs to try to gain more weigh than a woman who started her pregnancy overweight. Note that weight gain in the latter part of pregnancy seems to be more important because the fetus is growing so quickly.

Many women who lose weight in the early months make it up once morning sickness subsides. Some women do not lose weight at all, despite episodes of vomiting. However, becoming anxious about weight gain, or the lack thereof, simply generates more stress.

In understanding weight loss, you should be aware that different women have a wide range of total body water. About 57 percent of a woman's desirable weight before pregnancy is water if she's under 18 years old, and about 51 percent is water if she's 18 to 40 years old. An overweight person may have a smaller proportion of water in her body, because there is less water in fat tissue. This means that when a leaner woman loses weight, the percentage of water lost will probably be greater compared to an overweight woman who loses weight.

Some doctors consider hospitalizing a woman with morning sickness once her weight loss reaches 5 percent of her body weight, so a thinner woman may be hospitalized sooner than an overweight woman. These days, most intervention occurs in the obstetricians' offices because of cost containment pressures from insurance companies.

ICD CODES FOR HYPEREMESIS

What is interesting about data collection, especially for the ICD-9 codes for hyperemesis gravidarum is that the definitions do not include the words malnutrition or weight loss. (Recall from Chapter 4 that the International Disease Codes are used to track the worldwide incidence of certain diseases or conditions.) The National Center for Health Statistics lists five codes for hyperemesis:

643.0 Mild hyperemesis gravidarum starting before week 22 of the pregnancy

643.01 Hyperemesis gravidarum with metabolic disturbance, which includes dehydration, carbohydrate depletion and electrolyte abnormalities (such as potassium, phosphorous, magnesium) and starts before the end of week 22

643.2 Late vomiting of pregnancy, which includes excessive vomiting after week 22

643.8 Other vomiting during pregnancy due to organic disease or other causes specified as complicating the pregnancy

643.9 Vomiting as a reason for care during pregnancy; length of gestation unknown

The code for malnutrition is 263.9, and the code for weight loss is 783.21. Because multiple codes can be used to classify a person's condition, I asked a few obstetricians whether they put these codes in for their hyperemesis women, and several said "no." It seems almost impossible to think that a woman with hyperemesis wouldn't be malnourished! Perhaps a more comprehensive code should be considered.

MARGINAL FLUID CONSUMPTION

Most people have a daily fluid need of 2.5 liters (2.65 quarts). About two-thirds of the fluid requirement is obligatory—that is, it is the necessary and required amount of fluid needed daily to remove waste materials from the body in the urine. The body also needs fluid for the proper functioning of the gastrointestinal tract.

About one-third of the daily fluid you take in is lost through the lungs by breathing and through the skin as perspiration. To be safe, aim for 8 to 10 (8-ounce) glasses of fluid a day. A way to keep track is to plan to drink two-thirds of a cup of fluid for every waking hour, which may be a chore if you're nauseated. To make it seem more manageable, try for a shot glass every 10 minutes.

Normal fluid consumption for a healthy person comes from three basic sources:

1. Fluids ingested. This accounts for about 50 percent.
2. Foods consumed. Many foods contain a certain amount of fluid, and on average this accounts for slightly less than 1 quart.
3. Metabolism of food. Also called oxidation, this long, elaborate series of biochemical events releases small amounts of water in the process. The water generated from metabolism accounts for about 14 percent of the daily total.

Water in the body is critical to maintaining health for proper biological reactions to occur, to regulate body temperature, and to avoid constipation.

Choosing foods that contain plenty of water can prevent both constipation and dehydration. Table 10.2, in a later section, shows how small differences in food choices can make a big difference in maintaining hydration. Foods with more fiber also help to prevent constipation. Foods can lose water in preparation, such as by toasting or cooking.

CONSTIPATION

Four factors affect bowel habits:

1. Fiber content of the diet
2. Fluid consumption
3. Regular daily exercise or activity
4. Medication

The first two factors may be more obvious than the last two. Getting regular daily exercise, of course, depends on your overall well-being, which is certainly influenced by nausea and vomiting. Some medications designed to reduce the spasms in the stomach that propel food upward can also reduce intestinal peristalsis, the progressive waves of contraction and relaxation in the intestinal tract that move food through. When peristaltic action is reduced, intestinal matter moves more slowly than usual. The result is that more water can be reabsorbed from it, especially if fluid intake is low. Although this helps maintain hydration, the stool becomes harder and bowel movements can become difficult.

Even though prune juice doesn't have any fiber, it's great for stimulating the bowel and is often used to relieve constipation. You do have to develop a taste for it, however.

There are several new products out that will add invisible fiber to juices. One such product is called Benefiber, made by Novartis. I watched a demo where it was added to water, and you couldn't tell! For more information go to http://www.benefiber.com.

WATER AND FIBER CONTENTS OF SOME FOODS

Table 10.2 Water and Fiber Contents of Foods

Type of Food	Serving Size (average)	Water Content (in tbsp)	Fiber Content (grams)
White bread	1 slice	2	0.5
White toast	1 slice	1	0.6
Cracked-wheat toast	1 slice	1	1.4
Cracked-wheat bread	1 slice	1.5	1.3
Mixed-grain bread	1 slice	2.0	1.6
Mixed-grain toast	1 slice	1	1.6
Soda crackers	8 crackers	1	0.7
Apple juice	1/2 cup	8	0.1
Medium apple	2–3/4 in.	8	3.4
Milk	8 oz	16	0
Lemon yogurt	8 oz	8	0
Oatmeal (quick)	1 package cooked	6	2.0
Cream of wheat	1/2 cup cooked	7	1.7
Mashed potato	1/2 cup	5	1.5
Boiled potato	5 oz	5	2.0
Baked potato	7 oz (large)	9	4.7
Gelatin dessert	1/2 cup	7	0.1
Gelatin-carrot salad	5 oz	8	1.1

Poorly managed tension and stress can cause gastrointestinal (GI) problems ranging from diarrhea to constipation. When the muscles in the GI tract are relaxed, the contents are moved along normally; however, tension can disrupt this process. The tension can be as subtle as not having your own bathroom available on demand, for example, when you're away from home or you have house guests.

When you have a choice among foods, select the one with both the most fiber and most fluid, if possible. Table 10.2 gives water and fiber contents, based on serving size, for certain types of foods. The recommended dietary intake (RDI) for fiber is 25 grams per day. Some foods that are particularly high in fiber are stewed prunes, baked beans, almonds, and raisin bran cereal.

At times it may be difficult for you to find foods that contribute both fiber and fluid to your diet. Severe cases of constipation, requiring manual disimpaction by a doctor, have been caused by serious morning sickness. Because disimpaction can be uncomfortable, embarrassing, and expensive, prevention is the best approach.

ANEMIA

Most anemias during pregnancy are caused by low iron consumption or previous excessive blood loss through menstruation. When you're newly pregnant, iron deficiency can take on new significance if your consumption of protein foods is low. Your get up and go will feel like it got up and went! Check Table 10.3 for some foods that can help boost your iron content (some can also contribute to your fluid and fiber intake). The RDI for iron is 30 milligrams per day. Meat, especially red meat, is generally a good source of iron, but iron is also added to some cereal and grain products. Beans can also provide iron; for example, 1 cup of baked beans has about 5.04 milligrams of iron.

Table 10.3 Fluid, Fiber, and Iron Contents of Some Foods

Food	Serving Size	Fluid Content	Fiber Content(in g)	Iron Content (in mg)
Banana	1 medium	5 tbsp	2.3	.35
Apple	1 medium	8 tbsp	3.4	.25
Milk	8 oz	16 tbsp	—	.11
Broccoli	1/2 cup cooked	5.5 tbsp	2.0	.56
Carrots	1/2 cup cooked	6 tbsp	1.5	.48
Chicken	3 oz baked	3 tbsp	—	1.01
Lean pork chop	3 1/2 oz	3 tbsp	—	1.07
Calf's liver	3 1/2 oz	4 tbsp	—	6.8
Egg, cooked	1 medium	2 tbsp	—	1.04
Kidney beans	1/2 cup cooked	6 tbsp	6.4	1.7
Smooth Peanut butter	2 tbsp	1 tbsp	—	0.6
Swordfish, ckd	3 oz	3 tbsp	—	0.9
Enriched rice	1 cup cooked	8 tbsp	—	1.8
Brown rice	1 cup cooked	8 tbsp	CK	1.0
Prune juice	8 oz	7 tbsp	—	1.5
Total cereal	1/2 cup	—	1.0	9.0

Anemia often manifests itself as fatigue. Because of reduced amounts of iron, the blood can't carry as much oxygen to the body parts. Women, pregnant or not, who suffer iron-deficiency anemia are also less tolerant of cold. Getting adequate iron requires a concerted effort.

As a point of reference, the prepregnancy daily allowance is 15 milligrams of iron. For pregnant women, the daily allowance doubles to 30 milligrams per day. Most pregnant women take prenatal vitamins with iron or other iron supplements to prevent or resolve anemia. However, iron can be irritating to the stomach. Taking iron with food can reduce this problem, but if you're having nausea and vomiting, this may be difficult. Iron can also cause constipation, especially if fiber and fluid intakes are low.

If it's not possible to take an iron supplement every day, you should eat as many high-iron foods as possible. Although anemia may be a problem, most doctors and nutritionists believe it's most important to prevent dehydration first. Sometimes it's not possible to solve all the problems at once, and setting priorities becomes critical.

TOOTH AND GUM PROBLEMS

What you regularly eat affects the health of your teeth. High-fiber and high-protein foods don't contain many carbohydrates, which if left on or around the teeth allow mouth bacteria to produce acids that can erode tooth enamel. During morning sickness, the foods that are best tolerated may not be the ones that promote dental health. For a few days at a time your daily diet might include large amounts of crackers, rice, puddings, and yogurt drinks. It becomes even more important than usual to brush your teeth as frequently as possible to remove particles of sugars and starches. According to new observations, some dental researchers suggest waiting about 1 hour after vomiting to brush your teeth. Be sure to at least swish and spit to rinse your teeth off after a bout of vomiting.

Many women find that brushing their teeth can become a trigger for vomiting. The back and forth motion of the toothbrush can generate a premature gag reflex when it gets close to the back of the throat. The smell and taste of your usual toothpaste can also become a problem. Sometimes changing your toothpaste brand makes a huge difference. I like Tom's of Maine Ginger-Mint toothpaste. It hardly has a taste or smell and the texture is very smooth. Toothpaste with baking soda in it works well for some women.

If you can't brush your teeth, I suggest putting a small dab of toothpaste in your mouth and swishing it around with a big mouthful of cold water. Squeeze the water through your teeth as you spit it out. You need to protect your dental enamel as much as possible, especially if you are doing a lot of vomiting. Swishing and spitting is better than nothing.

If you can brush your teeth but can't handle the taste of toothpaste, just brush with water. To remove food particles in between your teeth, daily flossing is recommended. If you can't stand flossing right now, rinse your mouth several times a day with water. Because plain water is also high on the complaint list, try using naturally flavored water. For mint water, crush a handful of fresh mint leaves and put them into the bottom of a large glass bottle. Fill the bottle with cold water and refrigerate it. As water is used, replace it to keep the bottle full. Change the mint leaves every other day. For lemon water, slice a whole lemon and put into a large glass bottle. Follow the same directions as for mint water. Limes are another possibility, or try a combination of both.

If your gums are bleeding, be sure to let your doctor and dentist know. It could be because the vitamin C content of your diet is low. I asked my dentist if he can tell whether a woman has had bad morning sickness, and his answer was "yes." He can tell in the same way that he can tell whether a woman has a history of bulimia—dental erosion. He also said that dentists can apply extra fluoride treatments to teeth to help reduce the incidence of cavities.

In lieu of brushing your teeth, there's a new product on the market called Vitaball. It's actually a gum ball with vitamins in it. Chewing gum has been known to increase saliva, which helps reduce cavities. Vitaball also has some vitamin C in it, so trying this is worth a shot. Don't overdue the Vitaball, however, and be absolutely sure that any little kid in your household can't get into the Vitaball bottle, thinking it's candy. Take precautions with any and all medicines in your household, including vitamins and minerals, and always have the poison control numbers handy wherever you are. Check out www.vitaball.com for more information on this vitamin gum.

There are two small areas on the tongue that are referred to as the vagus nerve. The vagus nerve has connections in many places in the body, and one major connection is to the stomach. It may be that brushing close to these triggers nausea or a gag reflex.

Licking lemons or limes helps settle some women's stomachs (and lemons and limes contain lots of vitamin C and potassium). In addition, acidic foods have been reported to sharply increase the rate of salivation, which may lessen the possibility of damage to the dental enamel as a consequence of eating lemons and limes. At any rate, I've found that the period of lemon-eating is usually too short to be worrisome. If licking lemons reduces your incidence of vomiting, you're a bit ahead of the game.

IRRITATION OF THE THROAT AND NOSE

Women are bothered by the throat irritation that accompanies vomiting. As a result, they may select less scratchy foods, such as soft bread rolls. Many women report that orange juice is the most likely food item to be vomited through the nose, and they avoid it after the first occurrence. Eating the pulp from oranges seems to pose less of a problem. Eating ice chips seems to be a quick way to soothe a red, raw throat. Incidentally, historically, eating ice has been called pica. Ice is a different form of water, but we don't call drinking water "pica".

SALIVA

Many women complain that excessive saliva adds to their nausea. Saliva production is beyond conscious control. In fact, saliva normally bestows many benefits. It provides one of the first phases of the body's defense system because it helps to destroy bacteria in food. Saliva also helps to lubricate food, making swallowing easier. The production of saliva is controlled by the taste and smell centers of the cerebral cortex. Some medication given to try to control nausea and vomiting can also affect saliva production, which may influence a woman's unconscious choices of food.

Pregnancy hormones have been shown to change the composition of saliva enough to cause a difference in taste perception. Investigators have found that even distilled water can taste bitter. In the early weeks of pregnancy, women often complain that various foods "just don't taste the same anymore." Women are relieved to learn that an actual physiological change has occurred and that this perception is not psychological.

Tasting food has a lot to do with saliva. The flavor components of foods and beverages are dissolved in saliva, which then washes over the taste buds. Humans can taste salt at a ratio of 1 to 400, sourness at 1 part per 130,000, and bitterness at 1 part per 2 million. There is a protective message here. Because many of nature's bitter substances are associated with poisons, the ability to detect bitterness at this range was probably a matter of survival. Saliva is just another part of a survival scheme, although if at this point you are in the misery sequence of morning sickness, it may seem counterproductive.

Saliva contains the enzyme amylase, which is helpful in starch breakdown. One of the main components of saliva is bicarbonate, which counters the effect of acids produced in the mouth and stomach, such as lactic acid and hydrochloric acid, respectively. A high level of saliva with its corresponding high level of bicarbonate would also protect the teeth from the effects of gastric acid, another acid from the stomach, which comes in contact with teeth during vomiting. Saliva also contains calcium, an effective buffer that minimizes calcium loss from the teeth.

Some women with morning sickness experience excessive saliva, or what's know in the medicinal field as ptylism gravidarum, which basically means "a lot of spit by a pregnant woman." We found from a readers' survey done with Fit Pregnancy magazine, that 37 percent of the over 300 respondees commented on having excessive amounts of saliva. Perhaps women who are more likely to vomit produce more saliva as compared to those who suffer nausea only. It's also possible that the extra saliva is produced to neutralize the gastric acid from vomit in the mouth as well as to provide some measure of protection for dental enamel. However, dehydration, fear, and anxiety can reduce saliva production, as can some antinausea medications.

EARLY SATIETY AND OVEREATING

As difficult or impossible as it sounds, women with nausea and vomiting do overeat from time to time, generally between bouts of illness. Some pregnant women have a tendency to speed eat, and it takes time for the brain to appreciate the volume of food that is ingested when you eat quickly.

For the woman with morning sickness, speed eating can have deleterious consequences. Gastric distress may result in renewed episodes of vomiting. So, despite the internal signals that are being sent to hurry up and eat, it's important for a pregnant woman to take her time, chew slowly, and stop eating when she begins to feel the least bit full. If in a little while her hunger still persists and her stomach feels stable, she can have another small meal. Pregnant women need to learn to listen to their stomach messages and ignore pressure from family and friends to have just one more bite when the internal message is "enough!"

Other factors, such as fear and depression, can decrease gastric secretions and blood flow to the stomach, and this can delay stomach emptying. It's difficult to know how much worry and stress a woman with morning sickness is experiencing, which adds to the problem.

MUSCLE LOSS FROM PROLONGED BED REST

Muscle loss occurs with inactivity, especially prolonged bed rest. It is a case of use it or lose it: Muscles keep their tone only with regular use.

HEIGHTENED PHYSICAL DISCOMFORT

People who are dehydrated often can't tolerate extremes of temperature, especially cold. Turning up the thermostat when you feel cold only serves to hasten fluid loss through the skin. A better alternative is to wear one or two pairs of absorbent cotton or wool socks (or a cotton blend), cotton or silk long johns, and a long-sleeved T-shirt under ordinary clothes. And add a hat! Heat lost through the top of the head can amount to 40 percent.

Your choice of clothing also makes a difference in your overall level of comfort. Loose clothing permits a layer of air between the body and clothes to hold in warmth. Many pregnant women also find clothes that are snug around the waist annoying. If you're indoors, bundle up to be comfortable. Make sure that the clothes you add are loose and bulky, not tight and confining.

If you've lost weight, you may become chilled more easily, your body has lost some of its insulating layer of fat. When you feel cold, you may start to shiver. Shivering is actually an attempt on the part of the body to generate heat and uses up a fair number calories, so conservation of your body heat is important. Another physiological response to being chilled is a contraction of thousands of muscles on the sebaceous glands. These glands then produce an oily insulating secretion that is thought to help retain heat and water. Some women wonder why they feel so sticky just from lying around when they're sick, and this may be part the explanation.

You may find that breathing colder air is more comfortable, perhaps because it reduces the odors you can detect. However, if the environment is too cold, 68°F or less, the body uses more oxygen, and hence more calories, to produce heat. Several women have reported to me that a violent shiver in a cold environment, for example starting the car on a subzero winter morning, is enough to trigger a cycle of nausea and vomiting. If that turns out to be true for you, ask someone else to start and warm your car if possible.

Some women report that their skin seems extra-sensitive, making skin contact unpleasant. One universal sign that nausea is beginning to escalate is a desire to not be touched.

Spending several hours a day in bed between stale sheets can keep you from feeling rested. Change your sheets more often and try using pure cotton sheets. Cotton absorbs body moisture better than polyester-cotton blends, so these sheets may be more comfortable. Some women prefer scratchier surfaces on bed linens. If you air dry your sheets on a drying rack instead of putting them in the dryer, you'll be able to change the texture of most sheets. Experiment to see what works best. As far as bed linens go, women often say the highly colored ones have more of a chemical smell, so try white sheets.

You may feel more rested if your mattress is turned and rotated. This is something that bedding manufacturers recommend to extend the life of the mattress, but few people do it regularly.

SLEEP DEPRIVATION

How much sleep, on average, is lost due to morning sickness isn't known. We do know that inadequate sleep will wreak havoc with your psyche. Sleep deprivation is a common torture treatment during war time. We also know from rat studies that fed rats who are not allowed to sleep die faster than partially fed rats who get to sleep. When the body doesn't go into the delta phase of sleep, the stress hormone continues to do damage and the body has no time to repair itself. One study showed that 24 hours of sleep deprivation has been compared to the equivalent body alcohol level of 0.01 percent—the legal threshold for drunken driving.

VERY BAD MORNING SICKNESS AND PREGNANCY OUTCOMES

A comprehensive review of pregnancy outcomes and severe morning sickness or hyperemesis gravidarum is not a pretty picture. (More details about this will be given in Chapter 15, "Purple Heart Motherhood.") In a nutshell, four women lost their pregnancies spontaneously, probably as a result of severe malnutrition just before the 13-week mark. Three other women decided to terminate their pregnancies after 13 weeks of misery. There were six fetal losses, or miscarriages, by 18 weeks of pregnancy. In this group of women, the average weight loss was 13 kilograms, or an incredible 28 pounds. Of the entire group of 25 case reports that were analyzed, three quarters of women had problems postpartum including problems with vision, short-term memory loss, and difficulty walking.

SOME WORDS OF ENCOURAGEMENT

By now, you've probably figured out that this morning sickness misery has a lot of angles. Hopefully, this verse I penned years ago will provide just a little bit more emotional fortitude.

Holding On

Child of mine, you'll never know
What I went through to make you grow!

Time has always past with speed
Except for now—it's so slow indeed.

That my intake waxed and waned
What a struggle for a pound of gain!

Days of gloom and nights of pain
There were moments I'd gone insane!

Having children—a life-long goal.
It's not as easy as I'd been told!

When I see you by my side
I know that I will burst with pride.

That you flourished and developed fine
Oh precious dream—this child of mine.

Chapter 11

Worst-Case Scenario: Being Hospitalized

MIGUEL AND SONIA

Like David (from Chapter 10), Miguel was a second-time father. With the first pregnancy, he'd been surprised to find that morning sickness lasted as long as it did, because all the books about pregnancy that Sonia had bought said it should be over after the first trimester. His private concern about his wife's health and the baby's mounted with every passing day of her nausea. When the nausea finally ended after 5 months, Miguel felt as if a lifetime had passed.

With the second pregnancy, he expected morning sickness. His main concern every day was getting their 3-year-old, Ana, dressed and to the caretaker of the day. When Miguel and Ana visited Sonia in the hospital, where she was receiving intravenous nutrition, Ana clung to her father's pant leg, afraid of the tubes. She preferred to see the babies at the other end of the ward. Miguel said that visiting and spending time with his wife was impossible because he was always running after Ana. He admitted that the most difficult task he faced when Sonia came home was emptying her emesis basin.

Sonia finally decided she could no longer function safely at home, care for her active daughter, and battle morning sickness. The morning events before her admission included a verbal explosion at Ana, who had come running into the bedroom, and leapt on the bed with gooey fingers slathered with peanut butter and jelly. This was on a day when the baby-sitter called to report she was down with the flu and couldn't do child care. "Can't you understand I'm sick?" Sonia had yelled. Ana's bewildered face crumbled into a flood of tears, and she began to wail. Sonia thought, "I'm becoming a witch over this!"

The 400-bed community hospital Sonia's doctor was admitting her into had only one person working at the admissions desk. That afternoon was especially busy, with youngsters and elderly people being admitted with dreadful respiratory complaints—the big worry was that the respiratory problems were caused by SARS or pneumonia. Sonia sat conspicuously with a dainty, pink, kidney-shaped basin. She wondered who designed such inadequate items. Anyone who knows a hyperemesis woman should realize the current basin was clearly not deep enough. She also thought that there was no privacy factor with these basins and decided that a more useful receptacle would be one of the pink water pitchers she'd be seeing in a few hours at her bedside. A water pitcher at least would deep but, more importantly, it would have a lid for privacy. She didn't want the world to view her vomit if it happened.

After what seemed like hours of waiting, it was Sonia's turn. The gum-snapping receptionist sported a tongue ring, which Sonia noticed between chews. The thought of a tongue ring sent Sonia into small waves of nausea. But it was the witch-like false nails, clicking away on the computer keyboard that caused Sonia to elicit a tone that sounded like "arff." The receptionist stopped typing and shot Sonia a look that said "I dare you to throw up on my desk!"

A nurse finally took Sonia to her room in a wheel chair and said, "I'll bring your paperwork up." Minutes later, Sonia collapsed in tears on her hospital bed and told the nurse who was trying to admit her that she needed at least 20 minutes alone. It was all way too much for her. She's never read about any of these things in all her books about what to expect during pregnancy.

Sonia had a prolonged stay in the hospital because she had complications when her intravenous nutrition was started. Having starved for weeks before her doctor admitted her, she experienced *refeeding syndrome*. Although carefully monitored by the Metabolic and Nutrition Support Services, her obstetricians were not familiar with that particular situation and were worried about sending Sonia home with all the paraphernalia that was required.

Sonia described her problems with refeeding syndrome when her intravenous nutrition was advanced a little more aggressively than her debilitated nutritional state could tolerate. Her electrolytes (or blood chemistries) of phosphorous, magnesium, and potassium all dropped in the first day when her intravenous nutrition was started, and each electrolyte needed to be individually repleted. It was explained to Sonia that each of these electrolytes had an important role in the body—primarily in muscle contraction and relaxation. The most important organs that could be seriously affected were the heart and the lungs. The intravenous nutrition rate was dropped back while repletion occurred. In addition, Sonia's blood glucose rose to 160 milligrams/deciliter, higher than the goal of less than 90 milligrams/deciliter that the metabolic support team wanted to see. Additional insulin would have to be added to the intravenous solution.

Anticipating that perhaps blood glucose would be elevated after discharge, Sonia was taught how to prick her finger, draw blood onto a test strip, and use a glucose meter. Sonia was terrified of hurting herself, and it took several minutes each time she needed to position a spring-loaded lancet over her index finger to draw blood. She recalled her maternal grandmother had died of complications of diabetes, and now Sonia thought, "has this pregnancy given me diabetes, too?" Luckily, by the time Sonia was discharged from the hospital with her intravenous nutrition, her blood sugars had dropped to normal limits and testing was not required. The outpatient nutrition team followed her closely until 18 weeks, when her food intake picked up enough so that the intravenous nutrition could be discontinued.

Two years after the second pregnancy, Sonia and Miguel related all the details of their experiences to me while I was manning our Morning Sickness Booth at the Boston Baby Fair. Sonia asked some poignant questions about permanent birth control because she felt she could not risk another pregnancy. She thought having her tubes tied would be a great solution, but she'd recently heard from a medical report that tubal ligation increased the risk for ovarian cysts. And, although ovarian cysts can be painful and add another medical problem to Sonia's life, she couldn't help but think that it was the lesser of the two evils.

The high-risk pregnancy unit that Sonia had stayed in had a library because some women with complications ended up staying for weeks and months. Physically, they aren't necessarily as sick as the hyperemesis population, but they are pregnancy prisoners. Among the literary donations was a special edition of the New

Yorker magazine by one of the obstetrical residents. The July 5, 1999, edition was always delivered to the families of the HG patients (HGs as they are also known) so that what the patient experienced was seen as more universal.

This New Yorker edition was very special. One of the surgeon's I work with in Boston, now a very accomplished writer, writes the column "Medical Dispatch." This particular issue featured "A Queasy Feeling: Why Can't We Cure Nausea?" He described a woman named Amy and her horrific ordeal with a twin pregnancy. He was quite graphic with the mechanics of how one throws up. He described the whole scenario with one very poignant four-word sentence: "Her suffering was bottomless." Isn't that it in a nutshell!

HOSPITALIZATION

One goal of this book is to help women avoid hospitalization. This can be done by identifying a number of situations that can precipitate and aggravate nausea into unrelenting vomiting and possibly dehydration. On occasion, a hospital stay to correct dehydration is necessary. If this happens, morning sickness becomes known as hyperemesis gravidarum.

According to American statistics, about 1 pregnant woman in 72 is hospitalized with severe morning sickness. This means that each year about 55,000 pregnant American women require hospitalization, and, of those, about 40,000 are hospitalized due to dehydration. To prevent or delay hospitalization, some doctors perform intravenous hydration in their offices first. Other doctors' offices are either too busy or too small to provide this type of service.

The factors that affect your doctor's decision of whether or not to admit you to the hospital include the following:

1. *Amount of weight loss.* If you're seriously dehydrated and unable to eat, weight loss will be obvious. If you receive intravenous fluids, the scales will show an immediate gain of a few pounds. This is water weight; every 2 pounds reflects about 1 quart of fluid. If your weight remains significantly below your prepregnancy weight as the weeks go on, your doctor will be concerned.

2. *Amount of weight loss compared to your desirable body weight.* If you were slightly overweight when you became pregnant, your doctor may wait a little longer before hospitalizing you, as long as your blood pressure and urine output are adequate. An overweight woman has extra fat mass that can be used for energy. Because no one knows when the nausea and vomiting of pregnancy will end, the physician uses his or her discretion to admit patients or to wait.

3. *Fainting.* A woman can put herself and others at risk when she loses consciousness, even for a short time. Fainting is a sign of low blood pressure, resulting from low blood volume. This may be caused by vomiting or by inadequate consumption of liquids.

4. *Vomiting blood.* Vomiting blood may be caused by Mallory-Weiss tears, which occur when the tissues are torn where the esophagus and the stomach join. Dry heaves and violent and repeated retching can cause such tears. Vomiting blood can also be a sign of bleeding ulcers, which are life-threatening. A woman with a history of ulcers or gastritis may be more at risk for bleeding ulcers. Your physician needs to order tests to determine the cause and the significance of any vomiting of blood.

5. *Rib pain.* Violent retching and vomiting can strain rib muscles as well as facture ribs. The pain from broken ribs can make breathing and sleeping difficult. Hospital care for a few days should speed recovery.

6. *Jaundice.* When the skin begins to take on a green or yellow cast, jaundice may be the cause. Jaundice is a symptom of a variety of diseases, some major and some minor. Jaundice results when bile cannot be excreted in the usual manner. Pregnancy-related digestive upsets can disturb the normal functioning of the gallbladder and its ability to release bile. When bile is retained in the gallbladder longer than usual, the pigments that make up its greenish color can be absorbed into the rest of the body. Because jaundice is a warning sign of other potential complications, hospitalization, intravenous fluids, and observation are necessary.

7. *Physician's experience.* Before admitting a woman to the hospital, each physician exercises clinical judgment that depends on her or his previous experience with cases of morning sickness.

Even if your morning sickness seems quite severe, you may not need to be admitted to the hospital. But, should you be admitted, there are some things you need to know.

ADMISSION

If you're admitted through an emergency room, the process may be slow. Emergency rooms function on the premise that the biggest disaster comes first. A pregnant woman who is vomiting will probably be considered less of an emergency than a car-crash victim.

It's helpful if someone accompanies you and brings an "air sickness" bag and a few cold, wet facecloths.

If you're admitted through the labor and delivery rooms, the immediate needs of women in active labor will take precedence. Once the paperwork is finished, you'll be transported to a patient care unit by wheelchair or gurney. Many women with morning sickness are adversely affected by motion. Be sure that someone makes this fact known, or the ride may be one of the worst parts of your experience.

The attendant needs to know that (1) you're ready to vomit any minute; (2) you're highly sensitive to smells and the route needs to avoid the cafeteria, as well as anyone in the elevator bringing meals to patients; (3) sudden jolts to the wheelchair or gurney will make you instantly ready to vomit; and (4) you're somewhat claustrophobic and can't tolerate crowded places.

If you find that lying on your back on a gurney watching the ceilings go by gives you motion sickness, try staring at a stationary object and breathing deeply. If you smell disagreeable odors, hold a damp facecloth over your nose. (Sprinkle it beforehand with a drop of lemon or lime juice and carry it in a zippered platic bag in your handbag.)

A bad-aroma defense necklace can also help. Fold a large square bandanna diagonally. In the center place a squeezed-out wedge of lemon or lime or a few crushed mint leaves. If other natural fragrances have greater appeal, such as pine twigs, use them. Knot the scarf loosely around the lemon or mint and place the knot of the scarf at mid-chest, about eight or nine inches below your nose. You can bring the knot closer to your nose if necessary. Have your emergency necklace packed in your handbag in a plastic sandwich bag. I've found that when these kits are on hand, they're less likely to be needed.

ADMISSION INTERVIEWS AND QUESTIONNAIRES

On the patient floor, the assigned nurse will ask dozens of questions designed to help the staff take better care of patients, both physically and emotionally. Questions range from birth-control methods to food allergies. Sometimes a doctor's office makes copies of these questionnaires, which you can fill out beforehand at home. After an arduous journey from the admitting office to your patient room, you may not have the energy or interest to listen to these questions. If you are really wiped out, postpone as much of the admitting interview as you can. Just say, "I'm not well enough to do anything more right now. I'll do it later, after I get some rest." If the nurse seems insistent, it may be because the change of shift is coming up and these things are supposed to be done before someone else comes on.

If you're experiencing a high sensitivity to perfume or cologne, indicate on the questionnaire that their presence causes breathing difficulty. This is part of an effective defensive strategy. It's far easier to have a health provider put up a sign about your sensitivity to odors than for you to deal with visitors (and staff) individually.

THE EMPATHY FACTOR

The sad truth is that some people have empathy and some don't. Empathy grows with exposure to a variety of situations; some people are simply theorists. If you consider how long it took the medical community to take PMS seriously, you'll understand the uphill battle women with morning sickness face. Sometimes for health-care providers severe fatigue from overwork erodes the empathy factor.

Several ranks of medical people may be caring for you: The medical student, junior resident, senior resident, fellow, attending physician, nurse, care coordinator, and dietitian make up the team in most teaching hospitals. Each makes a contribution to care, and each can solve certain problems. For example, the nurse may put off taking your vital signs at 6 a.m. to avoid an abrupt wakeup. The dietitian may be able to reassign tray delivery if you find that a certain time is best. The resident may order that medications be crushed and mixed into applesauce if you strongly prefer them that way.

It may be helpful to keep in mind that, as advanced as medicine is, health-care workers can't necessarily fix everyone completely. Keep in mind, too, that hospitals today are being pushed to patch and dispatch patients as quickly as possible because of rising costs and pressure from insurance companies. With skyrocketing costs and insurance companies and medical plans requiring clients to pay a portion of the hospital bill, many people try to put off coming in for hospital care. This means that today's hospitalized patients are more acutely ill than ever before and often require more tests and procedures during their stay. That means more time and, in teaching hospitals, more required educational instruction, which leaves less room for general TLC.

MEDICATION

Often medication is prescribed that is intended to lessen nausea and vomiting, but it doesn't always work. It is also natural to wonder whether any of these drugs may have adverse effects on your baby. In a study sponsored by the National Institutes of Health, there were fewer pregnancy losses in two groups of women who took a variety of antinausea medications than in the group who took none. Somewhat different results have been found for laboratory animals, but it's unlikely that what is seen in one species of animal given large doses of drugs over long periods will occur in humans given smaller doses over shorter time spans. Any drugs used in pregnancy come under extremely tough scrutiny from many protective agencies and universities. Your doctor is the best source of advice in each individual case.

Bendectin was a classic case. The drug was used by more than 33 million pregnant women with severe morning sickness, in 21 countries, between 1957 and 1983. Although it was not shown in animal trials to cause birth defects, Bendectin was finally withdrawn from the market after a number of women whose infants had birth defects sued the manufacturer and were awarded large settlements. Most obstetricians believed the drug was not responsible.

Birth defects can be caused by a variety of factors, including family genetics; use of illegal drugs as well as some prescription drugs before and during pregnancy; exposure to lead preconceptually by both the mother and the father of the child; certain viral illnesses, such as measles and chicken pox; and bacterial infections. Also suspected in some cases is the advanced age of the father of the baby. In addition, exposure to toxic gases and radiation can result in damaged cells. There are some birth defects for which geneticists still do not know the cause. The range of reported birth defects, both major and minor, is about 2 to 3 percent overall in the general population.

Although the list of collective side effects of antinausea medications is extensive, the incidence of adverse effects is low. When any medication is required during pregnancy, doctors use the lowest dosage for the shortest period possible. If your nausea and vomiting don't abate—or even seem to get worse—during your hospital stay, your doctor needs to know. He or she will want to reexamine the type, dose, and timing of medications; the number of interruptions; the influence of roommate(s), including what they may be eating in your presence; and the generally capricious nature of nausea and vomiting. (Medications will be covered in greater detail in Ch 16.)

CARE IN THE HOSPITAL

The health-care team must try to figure out what the natural course of your case of nausea and vomiting is and minimize your physical and emotional discomfort. Hospital care can vary, depending on the size of the institution, the experience of the staff, and the number of unusual cases treated every year. You may become a patient on a gynecological floor, a maternity/postpartum floor, a surgical unit, or a medical unit in a private room, double room, or ward. A private room is worth its weight in gold, but you must be prepared to pay extra for it in many hospitals. Ask your doctor about ordering a private room as part of your care.

If your nausea and vomiting don't respond to standard management, a frustrated doctor may request that you be visited by a psychiatrist. The old notion that vomiting in pregnancy means an unwanted pregnancy and is a subconscious attempt to abort is usually the driving force behind this maneuver. However, meeting with a qualified psychiatrist can be a positive experience.

If you feel negative, remember that every woman has some ambivalence about pregnancy, and it's hard to be excited about having a baby when your life has come to a grinding halt. Many women begin to question their decision to be a mother.

Some women who suffer from severe morning sickness think about abortion, some women talk about it, and a certain percentage actually terminate their pregnancies. Women who resort to abortion often do so not because the pregnancy is completely unwanted but because the physical, financial, and mental stresses have overcome their capacity to cope.

PLANNING YOUR DIET

At some point in your hospital stay, a diet order will be written. It's best to work directly with the registered dietitian—ask for a consultation at the first opportunity. Depending on the hospital staffing and insurance, there may be a charge for this consultation. Discuss with the dietitian your food successes and failures. Ask what foods and beverages are available that are not listed on the menu.

As you've probably discovered, planning ahead for your next day's meals and snacks is just about impossible. Unfortunately, many hospitals are not set up like hotels. Requests for meal replacements and food changes can't be met instantly. Ordering several extra food items on each tray, labeling them, and keeping them in the closest refrigerator may be necessary. If a food doesn't require refrigeration, keeping it on your bedside table allows for a faster snack than going to a refrigerator, which may be down the hall. If you worry that the way the hospital's refrigerator smells or looks may escalate your nausea, ask your nurse to bring you the food. Many of the women

I've worked with prefer to see smaller trays with less food on them and to have snacks delivered between regular meals.

Ask if there's a way to call and get your requests changed if what you ordered doesn't seem to be what your palate wants. If canned shakes—or nutritionals, as they're called in the hospital—are available, try them. Be sure that they are ice cold and pour them into a cup. This lets the product breathe. Some women say they can smell the vitamins in them; other women enjoy them tremendously. If canned nutritionals don't become favorites, ask the dietitian to send cola or lemonade. (The small amount of caffeine in a cola beverage or an occasional cup of coffee shouldn't cause any problems.)

DINING WITH YOUR HUSBAND

If you want your husband to dine with you in your hospital room, ask to meet with the director of food services to find out how to arrange it. Be ready to pay up front with a check and get the details on how things work. (Keep in mind, however, that what your husband orders may not be something you'd like to see or smell if you're feeling sick.)

WORKING WITH DIETITIANS AND OTHER NUTRITION PROVIDERS

Dietitians know it's difficult, if not impossible, to talk about balanced nutrition with patients who are feeling sick. Women who are nauseated and vomiting report great stress because they can't eat properly. Eating a variety of foods from the recommended food groups is beyond their control, no matter how much nurses, doctors, and concerned family members and friends nudge. If the woman with morning sickness could eat better, she would. For any dietitians or other care providers reading this book, don't harass a pregnant woman about eating. If she's is interested in eating, then honor as many food requests as possible.

Most of the time, hospitals allow families to bring in requested food from home. If your food and beverage consumption is variable, the doctor or dietitian may start a calorie count, adding up everything you eat. But a calorie count may not take into account the calories lost if you vomit. Most women agree that asking about vomit is unpleasant. Saving it for the nurse to measure is even more revolting, although it's commonly done.

Another drawback of a calorie count is that it's a measure of the previous day's intake, which is ancient history. Continually being told that you're behind in your nutrients and calories can generate a fair degree of stress. Some women start to power eat, trying to consume more than is comfortable because they feel as if they're being scolded for misbehaving or for failing to cooperate. The result can be more vomiting, which leads to more stress and creates what feels like a downward spiral. Try not to let a calorie count add any more stress to your situation—it's simply a tool for the dietitian to use to spot trends.

If you're to improve your success rate with meals and snacks, you need to talk with the dietitian, understanding that she or he must address any specific doctor's order. If the doctor has ordered "nutrition consult, diet per patient's tolerance," you'll have an easier time negotiating about food. However, if the doctor trained with the tea, toast, and ginger ale crowd, it's going to be a little harder to get a cheese pizza if that's your craving of the hour. Some physicians want what they've ordered, and others let an experienced dietitian take charge.

Not every health-care provider has had extensive experience with or training in morning sickness, yours may be learning by doing. Renewed vomiting may or may not be related to a food you've been encouraged to eat. Just try to be patient. Remember that the people caring for you may be going by the books, and not all books have all the right answers! Try to discuss this with your doctor and your other health-care providers.

In earlier years, getting fluids or liquids into a woman to maintain a particular level of hydration and electrolytes was critical to survival. Nowadays, with intravenous fluids as a backup, doctors can start with solid foods. For some women, solids first and liquids later is far more successful in reducing the level of nausea and vomiting. Liquids can be added slowly to your routine once you've achieved gastrointestinal stability, or on your request. Keeping solids and liquids separate has been suggested by some books, but it's not an absolute rule. Whatever combination of solid and liquid food works for you should be used, whenever it works.

ARE YOU MALNOURISHED?

As you read in Chapter 10, there are criteria to determine whether you are malnourished. These guidelines don't just apply to the 70-year-old, homeless, bag of bones in the medical intensive care unit. These can be applied to you!

Personally, I think that the expanding waist line of the pregnant woman gets in the way of appreciating weight loss. If you started your pregnancy overweight, sometimes the thoughts are "with weight loss, there are fewer end-of-pregnancy problems, such as preeclampsia and gestational diabetes." And although that is somewhat true, there is only a certain amount of weight loss that should be acceptable. This is a very individual thing. Your prepregnancy weight situation, your weight loss, how long you've been sick, and how disabled you have become are all factors that come into play when interventions are being discussed.

SUPPLEMENTAL FEEDING
TUBE FEEDING

On occasion the doctor may discuss with you the option of tube feeding, especially if your food consumption is radically below your daily needs for days at a time. Although not the answer for every woman, tube feeding does provide nutrients, calories, and fluids. A thin tube is inserted through the nose, down the back of the throat and into the stomach. Tube feeding can make you feel a bit claustrophobic or anxious at first. Early in my career, clinical dietitians came from a neighboring cancer facility to demonstrate how to place feeding tubes, and I had the chance to experience tube feeding first-hand. A colleague of mine placed a tube in my nose, and I had the reciprocal opportunity. Although the tube didn't really hurt because of all the numbing spray that was administered beforehand, it was not a pleasant sensation. Having the tube in my nose made me feel anxious and caused me to gag a bit.

Some doctors allow you to try to eat with a tube feeding, whereas others prefer to wait a day or two. For some women who have the mostly nauseous end of morning sickness, this seems to work better than for women who have frequent problems with retching, vomiting, and gagging. Having food (i.e., formula) constantly dripping into your stomach sometimes reduces nausea. If the plastic tube in your nose is driving you nuts because of the smell, put some Vicks on it or maybe a minty lip gloss.

Before tube feeding is started, a care provider must take an x-ray to check the placement of the end of the nasogastric tube. (The amount of radiation needed to visualize the end of the feeding tube is miniscule but is of some concern to pregnant women.) The end position of the tube is critical. In rare instances, the nasogastric tube makes its way down the trachea, which leads to the lungs, instead of the esophagus, which end with the stomach.

Tubes have been inserted through the wall of the stomach and also further down in the jejunum to feed sick women. This is not something that health-care providers take lightly, and the risks and benefits are carefully evaluated.

INTRAVENOUS NUTRITION

If the hospital has a specialized service called nutrition or metabolic support, it may be possible to get special nutrients added to intravenous fluids for a short while, with or without the tube-feeding routine. The size and placement of the intravenous line will determine how many calories can be administered and what the nutritional contents can be. There are national guidelines for safe total parenteral nutrition (TPN). TPN generally will deliver 100 percent of a woman's needs within a week of starting. But some intravenous lines that go into an arm can't deliver 2,000 calories a day. Small arm veins can't tolerate the concentration of TPN without collapsing or getting very irritated. This is why TPN needs to run into a major blood vessel, where the blood volume can dilute the concentration of the solution. Smaller veins can handle peripheral parental nutrition (PPN), which can provide about 30 to 50 percent of a person's daily needs.

Central hyperalimentation (another name for TPN) uses the subclavian vein, which is next to the collarbone, rather than a vein in the arm, and completely bypasses the gastrointestinal system. Sometimes these feeding lines can be inserted in the middle of the arm and treaded up into a major blood vessel. There are several types of lines that last for certain number of days. I'm not going to bore you with a big discussion of this. If you happen to be in need of this, the team taking care of you will explain all you need to know. TPN carries a chance of infection and serious complications, so it is a last resort.

REFEEDING SYNDROME

One complication of tube or intravenous feeding is what Sonia had, refeeding syndrome. As you remember, there are electrolytes normally in the blood that come from the food you eat. When you don't eat, these electrolytes are markedly reduced. These electrolytes should be monitored and replaced by intravenous or oral solutions if they are low for any reason. Many of these important electrolytes are part of critical energy metabolic pathways, which keep the heart beating and lungs breathing, and are part of growing tissues. When nutrition is given too aggressively in the setting of low electrolytes, the electrolytes can drop further and put the patient in a crisis situation.

INVISIBLE FACTORS

Remember that when you're hospitalized many factors affect you that weren't present at home. However you are being fed, it's critical that you analyze the invisible factors that may contribute to nausea—smells, noise levels, the quality of your rest, and the number of times your sleep is interrupted. In addition, analyze the amount of motion you're subjected to. It may be anticipated or unexpected (like someone bumping into your bed), or visually experienced motion (such as television flash shots). Also consider the amount of stress and pressure you're undergoing, the level of hopefulness and optimism you can sustain under less than optimal conditions, and the amount of family and professional support you see and feel.

Figure 6.1, from Chapter 6, can help you organize this information. By recording this information, you can often identify a particular set or sequence of events that disturbs your equilibrium.

Figure 6.1

Time	Score 1–10	Level of Smells	Amount of Motion	Level of Noise	Preference/ Taste	Texture of Food Eaten	Quality of Climate

With that information in hand, preventive strategies can be considered.

If you're in a ward, your ability to fix things that bother you may be limited. The amount of change you can effect depends on your diplomacy and assertiveness. If you believe that the overall state of your health is declining instead of improving, and the invisible factors can't be controlled to your satisfaction, consider going home with hydration from a home-care company, if there is one in your area.

TIPS FOR COPING WITH HOSPITALIZATION

You may be dreading this ultimate catastrophe, being hospitalized, but women I've interviewed have told me that they were relieved when they were admitted, especially if they'd had a few long visits to the local emergency room for intravenous fluids. Remember, hospitals can be intimidating when you don't feel well, but they needn't be considered untameable monsters. You have the right to ask questions about options, and you also have the right to decline any particular treatment if you think it's not helpful. In addition, there are a number of things you can do to make your stay more comfortable.

OPTIONS FOR ADMISSION

Ask your doctor if being admitted straight from his or her office would be faster. Sometimes women are processed through the labor and delivery suites, the usual admitting office, or the emergency room. Each route has its snags and delays. Opt for the quickest and most dignified route. Tell your doctor ahead of time that this is important for you. Ask for a private room. Even if you think you can't afford it, imagine not being able to rest well because your roommate is up all night watching television, orders fish and broccoli at every meal, or is even sicker than you are. Even if you share a room with a postpartum woman, if she never experienced morning sickness, she may not have much sympathy for you. She may be busy showing her baby off and sharing her joy with the world, which is to be expected. Your doctor may not understand your desire for privacy, but don't be bullied or intimidated.

OBTAINING INFORMATION ABOUT YOUR TREATMENT

Ask your doctor if he or she will be there to start the intravenous fluids when you arrive. If not, ask who you should expect to see and how long after you arrive it will take to get your IV started. You may not be processed faster because you asked; hospitals operate on the principle of sickest first. But if you don't make your wishes known, nothing out of the ordinary will happen. If the intravenous fluid line is to be started by the IV team, you may not be able to get a specific name. Find out who the IV supervisor is and when the shifts change. Be aware that minor confusion and delays at the change of shifts are unavoidable.

If staffers are reluctant to provide specific information about your treatment, be sure you have available the name and phone number of the president and vice-president of the hospital. Call them directly if you must. Hospital administrators want satisfied customers and often will make sure you're tended to as promptly as possible. Remember, you're a paying customer! Hospitals also have patient representatives. Call the main switchboard operator ahead of time for these phone numbers.

THANKING YOUR CARE PROVIDERS

The IV nurse or technician is an important person. Because these staff members float from crisis to crisis and from floor to floor, they're not usually thanked regularly. I suggest that you ask your IV person for his or her name and then send a note of appreciation to the hospital president. You might also have a family member stash a few small boxes of chocolates in your tote bag as thank-you gifts to dispense during your stay. Chocolates are optional, but thank-you notes are vital.

RECORDING TREATMENT INFORMATION

Keeping a diary or log of your hospital experience may give you some sense of control. Ask how fast your intravenous solutions are running and when you should expect a new bag of fluid, and make note of this information. You might ask how to tell if something is going wrong. Does your IV site hurt? Ask who will fix it and when. If you're getting medication, ask about and note the side effects. Patient care units are required to have PDRs—*Physicians' Desk Reference to Phamaceutical Specialties and Biologicals*, which describes most medications given in hospitals—or an equivalent text. There are also hospital drug information hotlines.

Every hospital has a chief of service. If you find yourself without adequate answers, phone the chief of pharmacy directly. Keep in mind, however, that every medication has a purpose. Sometimes medication given brings temporary relief, and sometimes the medication is meant to break a cycle. In a few cases, adverse effects can occur. No one can predict what will be the case for any given individual.

Other health-care professionals that meet with you during your hospital stay are the maternity nutritionist or registered dietitian as well as the childbirth educator, if you're planning to take prepared childbirth classes. You might also want to meet the chaplain.

WHAT TO BRING

The more you bring to the hospital, the more you lug home. You'll want your address book. Hospitals provide "johnnies," the short back-wrap gowns, but you may feel better if you bring your own nightclothes, such as a knee-length, short-sleeved nightgown and baggy bloomer underpants. Most hospitals provide toothbrush, toothpaste, and soap kits, as well as shapeless green foam nonskid slippers. Don't bring any valuables, and mark your clothes ahead of time with an indelible marker. You may be cold because you're dehydrated; a shawl is probably a good idea, because it's loose and easy to put on and take off.

I recommend bringing two clean bras; four pairs of underpants; a fanny pack with your medical cards, driver's license, one or two checks, your favorite cosmetics, address book, and $10 or less (for newspapers and possibly gum from the gift shop); three pairs of white athletic socks; slippers; a nightgown; a shawl; hard candies; your own water, if you've found a variety you prefer; three boxes of assorted crackers (most hospitals only provide soda crackers); and a small plastic pail with a lid if possible (you may be sick away from your room, and although hospitals provide emesis basins, these are generally small kidney-shaped plastic containers without lids, which can be difficult to hold). Some women bring swimmer's nose clips to block disagreeable smells when they're trying to sleep. Earplugs might come in handy, because hospitals sometimes aren't as quiet as you might think. Sometimes hospitals buy budget-quality facial tissue, which can be rough or carry a particular scent. You might want to bring your own.

It's a good idea to bring your own pillow and a CD player with some of your favorite music. Bring enlarged copies of the signs in this book (from Chapter 6) to put on your door when you arrive. Bring a small roll of tape, too.

Bring a notebook. If you want to read, I suggest getting a large-print book from the library. Bigger fonts are easier to read.

Family and friends may send flowers. Some hospitals provide vases, but many don't. Consider bringing a mayonnaise jar. By the time you leave the hospital, most cut flowers will have lost their charm, and you won't want to drag them home with you. You'll hardly miss the mayonnaise jar, either. Some flowers are refreshing, whereas others are overpowering. Rubrem lilies are the worst! In my opinion, they are the smelliest flowers around.

Bring a small box of blank note cards, and write your hospital thank-you (or improvement) notes daily so you don't forget.

When You Go Home

When you're picked up at discharge, be sure to have someone evaluate how many cars are usually running in the area. Some hospitals have covered drive-up areas to protect patients from inclement weather. The downside of this is that car exhaust fumes are also trapped underneath, which can be extremely nauseating. If your husband (or whoever comes to fetch you) has to park in a nonregulation zone, be sure he puts a sign in the window saying "Emergency: transporting pregnant woman." Some hospitals offer valet parking; be sure the valet doesn't smoke in your car! Most pickup traffic is scheduled for midmorning, and it may be helpful to pick a different time of day to leave.

INSURANCE COMPANIES

Some insurance companies require that the patient call in daily to get an approval to continue coverage of hospital costs. Be sure to write down the first and last names of the people you talk with and exactly what they tell you to do. If you're asked for a doctor's letter, get it that day. Before you mail it, be sure you have a copy for your files. If you choose to read your chart, and you have every right to do so, a member of the hospital will be assigned to help you understand the terminology.

If you decide to leave the hospital before your doctor discharges you, or AMA (against medical advice), your insurance company may not pay for the visit. This scenario is rare, and generally insurance companies can't get their patients out the door fast enough. Some insurance companies will pay for home hydration therapy and some won't. Find out ahead of time what sort of coverage you have, because it may make a difference in your discharge care.

MAKING THE BEST OF A BAD SITUATION

If you've had a hospital stay and the experience has been helpful, sending a personal note sent to the hospital president can accomplish a great deal. First, it recognizes the efforts of your care providers. Second, it will bring attention to the misery women experience from morning sickness. Third, if you write down in detail both the most successful parts of your care and the places where improvements can be made, it will help the next woman who is admitted with morning sickness.

You might also consider making yourself available by phone to other women who must be hospitalized for morning sickness. Sharing your experiences can bring much comfort and can even speed advances in this area of health care.

Chapter 12

Recipes and Menus

LILLIAN AND ANDRE

Excited about his wife's first pregnancy, Andre never expected her to have severe morning sickness. He was surprised when, early in the pregnancy, he had to drive his wife, Lillian, to the emergency room of the nearby hospital for intravenous hydration. This treatment worked for one day. The second visit was an overnighter on the high-risk obstetrical unit. Here, Andre learned that Lillian's morning sickness might be short-lived or might last through the entire pregnancy. No one could tell him which queasy woman might have the long-term or short-term version of morning sickness. How was it that his dozens of aunts and numerous female cousins had never gone through this type of ordeal when they were producing all his relatives?

A two-income couple, Andre and Lillian had their lives carefully planned up until the unexpected challenges of severe morning sickness. If Lillian continued to be so sick, she would not be able to work. With the potential of losing one income, they needed to examine their financial situation. Andre found the anxiety of not knowing how it would all go incompatible with his expectations of a well-planned, comfortable life. They cut back on weekly expenses, such as health-club memberships, and sold her brand new luxury car—their second car—and bought a "budget-mobile" as Lillian came to call it. Morning sickness did not fit into Andre's life plan, and he found this very stressful. To reduce the number of trips to the grocery store once he returned from work, Andre invested in a cellular phone and called Lillian on the way home. He was never able to predict ahead what he might read on his cell phone's digital display. Messages ranged from, "KFC mashed potatoes x 2! Love you!" to "Wasabi sauce and fried shrimp from China Way on French. NOT CW on McCormack St! HURRY!"

FOOD OPTIONS

What and when you eat can make the difference between feeling miserable and feeling stable or at least "less worse," as many women say. Sometimes it's hard to plan out a whole meal's worth of food because you might be worn out. This chapter will give you several days of menus. Also, you'll find recipes to correspond to some of these foods. In gathering these recipes, I used the organoleptic approach discussed in Chapter 9—an approach based on our assessments of the physical and sensory attributes of food. See Table 12.1 for a list of food attributes.

Meals don't have to be huge—just eating something will help you recover. Change the size of the items in the meal depending on how you feel. Nothing is etched in stone!

Table 12.1 Physical and Sensory Attributes of Foods

Salty	Spicy
Crunchy	Liquid
Fruity	Hot
Sour	Tart
Smooth	Solid
Bland	Cold
Bitter	Tangy
Wet	Lumpy
Earthy/umami	Temperate
Sweet	Fizzy
Dry	

BREAKFAST

Day 1

Grapefruit half (add a tweak of honey on top if you like)

Shredded-wheat mini biscuits

1/3 cup slivered almonds

1 cup 1 or 2% milk (or plain or vanilla soy milk)

Cup of organic Earl Gray tea (by the way, tea is suppose to help with bad breath)

Day 2

Oatmeal made with 1% milk

1/2 cup strawberries on top

Raspberry tea

Dill pickle, if you need one

Day 3

Wheat germ mixed with peach yogurt

1 banana

1 cup of raspberry tea

Dish of ginger ice cream, if it works

Day 4

Scrambled egg with low-fat Munster cheese

Bran muffin

1 cup of calcium-fortified orange juice

Day 5

Cinnamon toast topped with small-curd, low-fat cottage cheese

Nectarine

Mint tea

Day 6

Bowl of cream of wheat with low-fat milk and topped with 1/4
cup chopped almonds and 1/4 cup cranberries

Cup of hot chocolate

Day 7

French toast made with cinnamon swirl bread

Regular maple syrup or Miriam's Ginger-Maple Syrup (see recipe)

1/2 cup of mixed fruit (try orange and grapefruit sections and add
some fresh cherries or grapes)

Ginger tea or plain tea with Miriam's Ginger-Honey (see recipe)

LUNCHES

With all your lunch meals, aim for at least one glass of water with lemon
slices or grapefruit peel added. Don't forget your fluid needs! You need
to get in 10 servings a day. It doesn't have to be all at once, however.

Day 1

Grilled cheese sandwich with tomato on whole-wheat bread

Baked apple with cinnamon and raisins (use nutmeg if you prefer
it to cinnamon)

1 cup of low-fat milk (if heated, add 1 tsp of ginger-honey)

Day 2

Roasted turkey breast in a whole-wheat pita pocket with cranberry sauce and lettuce

Spicy Fruit Soup (see recipe)

Dill pickles

Well-washed peach

Vanilla yogurt

Day 3

Bowl of minestrone soup

Whole-wheat crackers

1 or 2 slices Havarti cheese with dill

Day 4

Egg salad sandwich—1/2 egg and 1/2 tofu on oatmeal bread (or Extraordinary Noodles; see recipe)

8 oz raspberry or lime seltzer water or Lassi (see recipe)

2 oatmeal raisin nut cookies

Day 5

Standard grocery store tomato soup with 1 tbsp protein powder blended in before microwaving (in a big mug so as not to overflow while heating).

Directions will call for 1/2 volume of milk or water. Use milk if you aren't lactose intolerant or Lactaid milk if you are. Soy milk is an option if you are vegan.

Sesame bread sticks

1 cup of red grapes

8 oz of Spicy Ginger Ale (see recipe)

Day 6

Leftover whole-wheat spaghetti and turkey meat balls with pasta sauce

Spinach salad with cucumbers, radishes, and raspberry vingarette or Tangy Pear Salad (see recipe)

Dish of lemon sorbet or Cranberry Pudding (see recipe)

Apple-cinnamon tea

Day 7

Vegetarian bean burrito (organic and preprepared)

Chicken broth with lemon juice squeezed in just before serving
or Lemon Soup (see recipe)

Celery and carrot sticks (dip in dill pickle juice for 1/2 hr before
eating if you wish)

DINNERS

Day 1

Baked chicken (with fresh rosemary added to vinegarette marinade)

Baked potato with low-fat sour cream with chives

3/4 cup mixed vegetables

Coleslaw (prepackaged) with 1/4 cup raisins and 1/4 cup sunflower
seeds with a slaw dressing or 3/4 mayo mixed with 1/4 milk (flavors
will mellow if you do this at least 1 hour before dinner)

Smoothie: 1 glass low-fat milk blended with a banana

Day 2

Steamed salmon

Brown rice or Wild Rice Pilaf (see recipe)

Fresh string beans or Refreshing Asparagus (see recipe)

Sliced tomato

Dish of low-fat strawberry ice cream

Day 3

Baked potato stuffed with vegetarian chili and sharp Cheddar
cheese melted on top

Broccoli spears

Glass of low-sodium V8 juice

Fresh orange

Day 4

Brown-rice spaghetti with turkey meatballs and marinara sauce
or Cauliflower Walnut Casserole (see recipe)
Romaine lettuce with mandarin orange sections
Chocolate pudding
Glass of seltzer water

Day 5

Tofu stir fry with basmati rice or brown rice with lemon and
chicken casserole (see recipe)
Dish of frozen pineapple chunks
Glass of low-fat milk or vanilla soy milk

Day 6

Grilled lean steak
Red bliss potatoes
Julienne carrots
Asparagus stalks
Oatmeal raisin cookie
Glass of chai tea with milk

Day 7

Baked macaroni and cheese or Easy Cheesy Noodles (see recipe)
Green peas or Grapefruit-Cucumber Salad (see recipe)
Raw carrot and celery sticks
1/2 of grapefruit
Glass of lemonade

SNACKS

Whole-wheat crackers and cottage cheese
Chunky peanut butter in celery sticks
Air-popped popcorn
Mini rice cakes with almond butter

Granny Smith apple

Nectarine

Baked nachos with peach salsa

Pear

1 cup of red and green grapes mixed

Lemon yogurt

Chocolate milk

Packet of instant oatmeal made with milk

Potato Crunchies (see recipe)

Blueberry Soup (see recipe)

Peanut butter pudding (see recipe)

Banana Peanut Butter Power Shake (see recipe)

Quick Fruit Salad (see recipe)

Lime Pudding (see recipe)

There are two main questions to ask about whether a food or beverage is successful in ending a crisis: Is it (1) driving a thirst or (2) settling a queasy stomach? It's not surprising to find a woman going back and forth with choices.

RECIPES

CASSEROLES AND MORE

Brown Rice with Lemon and Chicken Casserole

(Earthy, tart)

Makes 4 servings

1 tbsp olive oil

1/2 cup finely chopped onion (about 1 small)

1 garlic clove minced

1 cup raw brown rice

2 1/4 cup fresh chicken broth

1/4 cup freshly squeezed lemon juice (or orange juice)

2 tsp grated lemon rind (or orange peel)

4 ounces chicken breast, cut into 1/4-by-2-inch strips

1/4–1/2 tsp of freshly ground pepper

Sauté onion and garlic in olive oil over medium heat. Add rice and chicken pieces and stir to cover. Add broth, juice, rind, salt, and pepper if you choose. Bring to a simmer, cover, and reduce heat. Allow to simmer for 45 minutes or until liquid has been absorbed and rice is done and fluffy. Garnish with freshly chopped parsley or sautéed almond slivers if you choose.

Cauliflower Walnut Casserole

(Earthy)

Makes 4 large servings

This is my favorite recipe and is used with the permission of two creative women, Linda Hackfeld, R.D., M.P.H., and Betsy Eykyn, M.S., who wrote Cooking a la Heart (available from Appletree Press, Good Council Drive, Suite 125, Mankato, MN, 56001).

Some women have reported that a plate with a lot of colors can increase their nausea—they prefer light, white, and tan foods during this time. Have someone make this dish for you, because preparation time is somewhat long. When you reheat, use low heat.

1 medium head cauliflower, broken into florets

1 cup low-fat plain yogurt

1 cup shredded cheddar cheese

1 tbsp flour

2 tsp low-sodium chicken-flavored bouillon granules

1 tsp dry mustard

1/3 cup chopped walnuts

1/3 cup dry bread crumbs

1 tbsp margarine

1 tsp dried crushed marjoram

In a medium-sized saucepan, cook cauliflower in water, drain, and put into 10-by-6-inch baking dish. Mix yogurt, cheese, flour, bouillon granules, and mustard and pour over cauliflower. Mix walnuts, bread crumbs, margarine, and marjoram together and sprinkle on top. Bake for about 20 minutes in an oven preheated to 400°F.

Easy Cheesy Noodles

(Bland)

Makes 4 servings

This recipe is used with permission of Nancy Clark, R.D., MS, from her book, Nancy Clark's Sports Nutrition Cookbook. I like this recipe for its versatility. Adding 1/2 cup diced tomato, 1/2 cup freshly chopped and cooked broccoli, and 1/2 cup al dente julienne carrots makes this a more nutritious and very colorful dish.

8 oz dry egg noodles

1 tbsp olive oil

6 oz low-fat cheese (munster for a blander meal, blue cheese or sharp
    cheese for tangy taste)

Optional: salt, pepper, dried mustard, parsley, garlic powder, Italian seasoning, diced tomatoes, steamed broccoli, peas, julienne carrots

Cook noodles according to package directions and drain. Add oil, cheese, and other ingredients of your choice.

Extraordinary Noodles

(Tangy)

Makes 4 large servings

12 oz of pasta noodles (vary the shape for interest)
1 1/2 tbsp poppy seeds
1/4 cup canola oil margarine
1/2 tsp ground nutmeg
1 tsp freshly grated lemon rind
1/2 tsp salt
Pepper to taste

Cook pasta in salted water as directed on package. Drain and keep hot. Toast the poppy seeds by placing them in an ungreased pan over medium heat. Stir or shake often for 5 to 10 minutes. Let cool for 1 or 2 minutes. Blend margarine, nutmeg, lemon rind, and toasted poppy seeds in small bowl. Toss all ingredients in warmed serving dish and serve immediately.

Gingered Butternut Squash

(Spicy, hot)

Preheat oven to 350ºF. Use the big end of one butternut squash and cut in half. Put 1 teaspoon of soy margarine and 1 tablespoon of ginger jam in each half. Place squash into a baking dish filled with hot water and bake for 1 hour. Remove from oven and serve.

An alternative method is to peel and chop up the solid end of the squash into 1-inch cubes, boil in small amount of water. To serve, put 2 tablespoons of ginger jam and 1 tablespoons of soy margarine in a coffee cup and heat in microwave. Drizzle over the squash and toss before serving.

Gingered Carrots

(Spicy, crunchy)

1 lb organic carrots, peeled and sliced lengthwise

2 tsp organic soy margarine

1 tbsp ginger jam

Because ginger has a reputation of helping to quell the queasies, try this easy recipe. Sauté the carrots on medium heat in a standard frying pan, turning them frequently until they look slightly browned. Turn the heat down to low and put the lid on for about 1 minute. Add in the ginger jam and stir until all the carrots are coated. Turn off the heat but leave the pan on the stove for 5 minutes. Eat either hot or cold.

Noodle Kugel

(Bland, crunchy)

Makes 8 servings

1 lb of cooked noodles

16 oz of low-fat cottage cheese

4 eggs, or equivalent egg substitute

1 cup low-fat plain yogurt

1 cup golden raisins

1/2 cup brown sugar

4 tbsp melted margarine

1 1/2 tsp vanilla extract

1/2 tsp cinnamon

Combine all ingredients in a pregreased oven-safe dish. Refrigerate overnight. Top with 1 tablespoon margarine and sprinkle with cinnamon. Bake in an oven preheated 350ºF oven for 1 1/2 hours, or until golden brown on top.

Refreshing Asparagus

(Tangy)

Makes 4 (3-stalk) servings

1 bunch fresh, young light-green asparagus

1 tbsp canola oil margarine

3 tbsp lemon juice

Trim woody ends off asparagus. Place in ceramic microwave dish with 1 tbsp water and cover with glass top. Microwave on high for 45 seconds or until crisp-tender. Melt margarine in microwave in a ceramic coffee cup with the lemon juice. Pour over hot asparagus and serve immediately.

Rice-Carrot Casserole

(Bland)

Makes 8 servings

2 cups partially cooked white or brown rice (start with 1 cup raw)

2–3 raw carrots

1 large onion, chopped

1 clove garlic, minced

2 eggs beaten, or equivalent in egg substitute

2–3 tbsp canola oil

2 tsp salt

1/4 cup dry skim milk powder

Preheat oven to 350ºF. Stir all ingredients together and pour into an oiled 7-by-7 pan and bake for 45 minutes to 1 hour. Add 1 cup of grated cheese to hot topping if desired.

Special Rice

(Hot)

Makes 4 (3/4-cup) servings

This is a great way to reintroduce milk into the diet after a bout of sickness. It's also good for people who hate milk or who are marginally lactose intolerant.

Sometimes milk can taste or smell to a pregnant woman like the cardboard carton it comes in. The solution is to buy milk in glass or plastic bottles. Don't store milk next to the onions in the refrigerator, either.

Cook 1 cup of rice slowly in 2 1/2 to 3 cups of low-fat milk until the rice is soft. Stir often and add small amounts of water if the milk is absorbed before the rice is tender. Serve hot or cold. Or add extra hot milk and cinnamon and eat like a porridge any time of the day.

For a change of pace, try fragrant Basmati rice or add 1 or 2 drops of vanilla or lemon extract during the final phase of cooking.

Wild-Rice Pilaf

(Earthy)

Makes 6 (1/2-cup) servings

2 cups strong chicken broth (preferably homemade)
1 small finely chopped onion
1 clove of garlic, chopped or crushed in garlic press
1 tsp finely minced fresh lemon rind
1 cup wild rice
1/2 cup brown rice
2 tbsp toasted sesame seeds

Heat 1 cup broth in large saucepan. When it boils, add onion and garlic, cooking until soft. Add lemon rind and both rices, along with the rest of the broth. Reduce heat and simmer for 1 to 1 1/4 hours or until rice is just tender. (You can also put the mixture in an oven-safe covered dish and bake for 1 hour.) Just before serving, stir in sesame seeds.

SALADS

Carrot Raisin Salad

(Crunchy)

Makes 4 servings.

1 cup grated carrots
1 1/2 tbsp raisins
1 tbsp lemon juice
1 tbsp mayonnaise
1/2 cup of sunflower seeds.

Mix all ingredients together and chill.

Cole Slaw Variations

If crunchy is a texture you like, consider the variations from grocery store slaw, or more properly called cole slaw, which simply means a salad of thinly chopped cabbage.

First: Take the premixed slaw out of the bag and soak it for 10 minutes (or more) in fresh water. Stick it in your salad spinner and dry.

To container #1: Add 2 tablespoons each golden raisins and sunflower seeds and 2 tablespoons (or more if you like) ranch dressing. Toss and let rest 1/4 hour before eating.

To container #2: Add a few tablespoons of dried cranberries and toss with a few tablespoons of raspberry vingarette. (Pack in lunch bag to eat at work).

To container #3: Add 1/4 cup of slaw dressing, 1 cup fresh spinach shopped into same size pieces, and 1 tomato diced. Add ground fresh pepper if you like.

To container #4: Add 1 diced up Granny Smith apple and 2 tablespoons walnuts. Toss with 1 tablespoon canola oil and low-sodium rice wine vinegar.

Cranberry Salad

(Crunchy, tart)
Makes 8 servings

1 cup whole cranberries
1 pkg lemon JELL-O
1/2 cup hot water
1 cup crushed pineapple

1 cup pineapple juice (drained from the crushed pineapple)
1 cup chopped celery
1/2 cup chopped walnuts

Dissolve JELL-O in hot water using half of the water specified on the package in a large ceramic bowl. Chill until partially set. Crush cranberries slightly with a potato masher if you have one. If not, put them in a zipper-sealed plastic bag and crush with a cookbook. Combine cranberries, pineapple and juice, walnuts, and chopped celery with the partially set JELL-O. Chill until firm.

Grapefruit-Cucumber Salad

(Tart)

Makes 4 servings

1 large cucumber, sliced thin (about 1 cup)
2 peeled large grapefruit or 3 cups grapefruit sections
2 tbsp canola oil
2 tbsp cider vinegar
2 tbsp sugar (or to taste)
1/4 tsp fresh dill

Toss all ingredients together in large bowl. Serve on chilled plates.

Grated Finnish Vegetable Salad

(Bitter) makes 8 servings (1/2-cup)

Vegetables:
1 cup grated carrots
1 cup grated rutabaga or white turnips

1 cup grated raw beets

1 cup grated apples

1 cup grated red or green cabbage

Mix ingredients together and arrange on a large plate.

Dressing:

1/4 cup freshly squeezed lemon juice

1/2 cup orange juice

1 tsp canola oil

1/4 cup chopped parsley

Mix together and pour over vegetables.

Quick Fruit Salad

(Tangy)

Makes 4 (1/2-cup) servings

1 peeled and sliced kiwi fruit

1 cup hulled fresh strawberries

1 cup grapes, black or green (or mixed)

8 oz plain yogurt

1/4 cup freshly squeezed lemon

1–2 tsp freshly grated lemon peel (well washed and scrubbed lemon)

Mix all fruit together. Mix yogurt and lemon juice and peel. Toss fruit with yogurt. Refrigerate any unused portion. (Or blend yogurt and kiwi in blender, add rest of fruit, and freeze in Popsicle molds.)

Tangy Pear Salad

(Pungent)

Makes 4 servings

2 fresh organically grown pears, thinly sliced (leave the peel on)
1 cup seedless red or green grapes
3 tbsp coarsely chopped walnuts
2 tbsp honey or Lyle's Golden Syrup
2 tbsp fresh lime juice
1 tbsp canola oil
1 tsp poppy seeds (or sesame seeds)
1/8 tsp salt
1/8 tsp ground allspice

Combine pears, grapes, and walnuts. Toss with remaining ingredients. Serve on romaine lettuce. Add 1/2 cup cottage cheese to each serving if desired.

Waldorf Salad

(Crunchy, tart)

Makes 4 servings

4 medium-sized tart, red apples with peels, cored, and diced
3/4 cup firmly chopped celery, well washed with vegetable brush beforehand
1/2 cup coarsely chopped walnuts
2/3 cup calorie reduced mayonnaise or plain yogurt
Add sprinkle of cinnamon or nutmeg if desired

Stir all ingredients together. To hold mixture together, add more yogurt as needed. Cover and chill for at least 2 to 3 hours. Serve on lettuce.

Walnut, Cranberry, and Celery Salad

(Crunchy, earthy)

Makes 4 servings

In a metal or ceramic bowl, mix 1 package of gelatin dessert, according to directions, with hot water. Mix in 1 cup diced celery and 1/2 cup chopped walnuts with 1/2 cup dried cranberries. Cover and refrigerate.

SOUPS AND PORRIDGES

Blueberry Soup

(Fruity)

Makes 6 (2/3-cup) servings

2 pints washed blueberries

3 cups water

1/4 cup sugar (or to taste) 1 1/2 tbsp potato starch

1/4 cup cold water

Put blueberries and 3 cups water into medium saucepan, bring to a boil, reduce heat and simmer for 10 minutes. Do not boil. Season with sugar and remove from heat. Mix potato starch with water, making smooth paste. Slowly pour into mixture, stirring constantly with whisk. Bring to a quick boil and remove from heat. Serve warm or cold, with or without sugar sprinkled on top.

Honeydew Soup

(Tangy)

Makes 4 (3/4-cup) servings

1 large honeydew melon
1 tbsp canola or soy margarine
3 tbsp minced onion
Salt and pepper to taste
2 tbsp chopped mixture of chervil, chives, and parsley

Seed melon and cut into large chunks. In medium saucepan, heat margarine and sauté onion until soft. Remove from heat and stir in melon cubes. Add salt and pepper if desired. Puree mixture in blender or food processor and refrigerate several hours or overnight before serving. Garnish with herb mixture. Serve cold.

Indian Rice Porridge

(Bland)
Makes 6 (1/2-cup) servings

3 cups low-fat milk
1 cup Basmati rice
1 medium egg
1/3 cup sugar (or less)
1/4 tsp salt
1/4 tsp almond extract

Put 2 cups of milk into medium saucepan and add rice. Cook slowly until liquid is almost absorbed. Beat egg into the remaining 1 cup of milk and add sugar. Add egg mixture slowly to mixture in saucepan, stirring constantly. Add extract. Serve hot or cold.

Lemon Soup

(Sour)
Makes 6 (2/3-cup) servings

4 cups water
1/4 cup golden raisins
1/4 cup sugar (to taste)
1 cinnamon stick
3 tbsp barley flour or potato starch
1/3 cup cold water
Juice of 1 or 2 lemons, or more if desired

Put water, raisins, sugar, and cinnamon in saucepan and bring to a boil. Cover and simmer 10 minutes, then remove from heat. Mix flour or starch slowly with cold water, making smooth paste, and add slowly to above mixture, stirring with whisk. Reheat about 10 minutes and discard cinnamon stick. When soup has thickened, remove from heat and stir in lemon juice. Serve chilled, with or without sugar sprinkled on top, or with whipped cream or yogurt.

Spicy Fruit Soup

(Spicy)
Makes 6 (8-oz) servings

2 medium oranges, peeled and cut into sections
1 medium peach, or 2 canned peach halves in light juice
1 large nectarine
1/2 cup lemon juice
1 tbsp orange juice concentrate
5 tbsp sugar

2 tsp cornstarch

3 cups orange juice

Pinch of salt

2 sticks of cinnamon

1/4 tsp ground cloves

2 tbsp flour

Optional: thinly sliced orange for garnish

Place chopped orange sections in bowl. In another bowl mix chopped peach and nectarine. Toss with 2 teaspoons of the lemon juice. Set aside. In a large saucepan, combine sugar and cornstarch. Gradually add orange and remaining lemon juice, salt, and spices. Bring liquid to a boil over high heat, stirring for about 1 minute. Reduce heat and continue to simmer for 5 to 10 minutes. Add chopped peach and nectarine to liquid and simmer again for 5 minutes. Remove pan from heat and allow to cool about 30 minutes. Add reserved chopped orange sections. Refrigerate several hours or overnight before serving. Garnish with orange slices if desired.

SNACKS AND DESSERTS

Cranberry Pudding

(Sweet)

Makes 6 (2/3-cup) servings

4 cups cranberry juice

1/2 cup sugar or honey to taste if using unsweetened juice

1/4 cup potato starch

1/3 cup cold water

Put juice (and sugar if used) into saucepan and heat, but do not boil. Mix potato starch slowly with cold water to make paste and pour slowly into juice. Stir well with wire whisk. Simmer pudding until thickened and translucent. Remove from heat. Sprinkle with sugar if desired and serve chilled. Add whipped cream or yogurt if you wish.

Easy Refrigerator Pie

(Cold, smooth, spicy)

1 package of vanilla instant pudding
12 oz of fat-free evaporated milk
15 oz of pumpkin pie filling
1 tsp pumpkin pie spice

Beat the pudding and the milk in a big bowl and refrigerate for 5 minutes. It will become thicker. Then stir in the pumpkin pie filling and spice. Pour into a graham cracker pie shell and refrigerate 1/2 hour. (Use a preprepared graham cracker crust pie shell for this recipe and save yourself an hour in the kitchen, or you could try making this with the Gingersnap Pie Crust recipe.) Or, if you don't want to have a pie, you can pour the pudding into eight refrigerator dishes and have high-calcium pudding instead.

Flan

(Bland, smooth)
Makes 6 servings

1 3/4 cups sugar
6 eggs or equivalent in egg substitutes or half and half
2 cups milk

1 tsp vanilla

1/4 tsp cinnamon

Preheat oven to 350°F. Place 1 cup sugar in the bottom of a glass pie plate and place in oven for about 20 minutes, or until sugar is caramelized. Remove from oven and cool to room temperature. Beat eggs with remaining sugar and gradually beat in milk. Add vanilla and cinnamon. Stir well.

Put pie plate with the caramelized sugar in a large pan, filled with 1/2-inch warm water. Pour the egg-milk mixture over caramelized sugar. Bake in preheated oven at 350°F for about a half hour. Cool to room temperature. Invert onto shallow dish.

Flowerpot Bread

(Earthy, crunchy)

2 cups unsifted whole-wheat flour

1 cup coarsely ground crushed wheat (if you can't find crushed wheat, you can use 1 cup of uncooked, old-fashioned oatmeal)

2 tsp baking soda

1 tsp salt

1/2 cup low-fat milk

1 tbsp honey

2 cups of plain yogurt

1 cup of walnuts (or you can add 1 cup raisins if you prefer)

Preheat the oven to 350°F. Mix whole wheat flour, crushed wheat, baking soda and salt in a big bowl. Add walnuts. Warm milk and honey so honey dissolves. Remove milk from stove and mix in the yogurt. Add the wet ingredients to the dry ingredients and stir well. Mixing must be quick or you will end up with a bread that might double as a brick! Pour batter into greased baking pans, or into a greased, clean juice can. Bake at 350ºF for 1 hour. If you use a juice can, use a can opener to remove the bottom of the can, after the bread has cooled, and push it out.

The original baking container for this bread is really a brand new clean terra cotta flower pot! Because we don't know whether flower pots contain lead that might leak out of the container, use the standard 4-by-4-by-7–inch bread pan or use a clean juice can. This recipe is modified from the original in a cookbook I bought on my first trip to South Africa, during which I interviewed both Xhosa and Zulu women about morning sickness. None of the tribal women I interviewed ate this Cape Dutch recipe, but it's a fun recipe to make and will get more fiber into your diet.

Gingersnap Pie Crust

(Crunchy, spicy)

1 1/2 cups of crushed gingersnaps
6 tbsp melted canola margarine
1/4 to 1/2 cup of confectioners' sugar

Mix all together and press into a 9-inch glass pie plate. You don't have to prebake this crust if you are going to fill it with the above mixture, however you need to chill it for 1 hour before you use it, or the filling will disintegrate the crust.

If you want to save time, you can bake it first, for about 10 minutes. Be sure its cooled off before you will it with a filling. Fill the crust with the filling in the Pumpkin-Cheese Pie recipe and bake the whole thing for 1 hour.

Ginger Sundae

(Hot, spicy, cold, smooth)

2–3 tbsp ginger jam
1/2 cup vanilla ice cream

This recipe could not be easier and it's really yummy. It was an invention for a very sick friend in early January 2004, one of the coldest winters of record in the northeast.

Take about 2 to 3 tablespoons of ginger jam, put it in a microwavable dish, and zap it for about 10 seconds or until it is bubbly. Then pour it over 1/2 cup of your favorite vanilla ice cream. Voila! This combination could be described as hot, spicy, cold, and smooth.

Can't find ginger jam? Don't fret. You can make your own! Take 1/2 cup of crystallized ginger. You'll find this in the baking section of most grocery stores. It's also known as Baker's Ginger. Chop it into small bits. Use a microwave dish and add 1/4 cup of water. Cover. Microwave about 30 seconds, or until it gets gooey. Vary the amount of water until you find a consistency you really like. Some women might want a ginger syrup and some a more solid, jam-like product.

Lemon Mousse

(Smooth, tangy)
Makes 2 servings

If you like lemon you'll probably love this world-famous lemon mousse. I refer to the texture of this mousse as a "solid liquid." It's a favorite among my patients.

Make a small package of lemon gelatin according to directions. Let it set up in refrigerator. Put 1 cup of the gelatin into blender, followed by 1/2 cup hard vanilla ice cream. Whirl for about 10 seconds, or until color is blended.

Lime Pudding

(Tangy)

Makes 4 (1/2-cup) servings

For a change, use lemon instead of lime.

2 tbsp sugar
1 1/2 tbsp cornstarch mixed with equal amount cold water
1 tsp margarine
1/4 cup lime juice
4 oz evaporated skim milk
4 oz plain yogurt
1 1/2 tsp freshly grated lime rind

In saucepan over medium heat, mix first five ingredients. Cook slowly, stirring frequently, until thickened. Remove from stove and pour into chilled oven-to-freezer baking dish. When cooled, stir in last ingredients. Serve immediately.

Miriam's Gluten-Free Gingerbread Pudding

1 cup Dutch Ginger Loaf (see page 306 for product information)
2 eggs
1–2 tbsp sugar or honey
2 cups milk
1 tsp vanilla

Preheat oven to 350ºF and put in a 9-by-9-inch baking pan of hot water filled halfway. Cut up 1 cup ginger loaf cake into 1/2-inch-size cubes. Divide these between two custard dishes.

In a small bowl, beat 2 eggs with 1 to 2 tablespoons of sugar or honey. Add 2 cups of milk to this egg mixture and a 1 teaspoon of vanilla. Beat the mixture with an egg beater or mixer just until blended. Pour over the gingerbread cubes and let soak for 10 minutes. Put custard dishes into hot water and bake for about 60 minutes. Carefully remove the hot water pan and custard dishes from the oven. Take the custard dishes out of the hot water pan and cool before refrigerating. Eat either hot or cold within 2 days.

If you are allergic to cow's milk, make this with plain soy milk with vanilla added or with vanilla soy milk and omit the vanilla flavoring. Each serving (which is pretty substantial—1 cup) will provide about 15 grams of protein. If you want to divide the ingredients into four custard-baking dishes, you can easily do so. Each serving would provide about 7 grams of protein. Baking time is reduced to about 45 minutes.

Orange Pudding

(Tart)

1 packet instant vanilla pudding
1 can (11 oz) of drained mandarin oranges

Even women with limited culinary talents and cooking space can make this recipe. It's actually one small children can help assist preparing. The original, using dried milk and water, came from a camping cookbook. Camp cooking books are creative aids to put variety into your eating life. Check out some books from a local library.

Prepare 1 packet of instant vanilla pudding with milk per instructions on the package. To this mixture, add one 11-ounce can of drained mandarin oranges. Stir well and refrigerate for 1 hour.

You can vary the fruit. Try drained diced peaches or pears.

Peanut Butter Pudding

(Earthy)

Makes 4 (3-oz) servings

1 1/2 tbsp chunky peanut butter

8 oz evaporated skim milk

1 egg plus 1 egg white

1/4 tsp vanilla

Blend all ingredients together until smooth. Place four small ramekins in a large baking dish that has been filled with 1 inch of hot water. Pour mixture evenly into ramekins and bake at 350ºF for about 45 minutes. Carefully remove from oven and cool.

Potato Crunchies

(Crunchy)

Makes 2 (1/2-cup) servings

Peel a large potato and shred in food processor. Put into a strainer and rinse with cold water. Pat dry with paper towels. Actually, you don't have to peel the skin off. You can use the whole thing—skin and all. However, if you choose to save yourself the time and energy of peeling, be sure you buy organic potatoes and scrub the skin with a vegetable brush thoroughly. This will greatly reduce the amount of natural pathogens inherent in the soil that may be left on the potato skin. Heat conventional frying pan coated with small amount of canola-oil cooking spray. Add potato shreds and sauté until brown and crispy. Season as you choose with salt, pepper, parmesan cheese, or vinegar.

A word about nonstick frying pans: I've heard bits and pieces about their instability after a number of uses. At this time, I'm limiting my own use with these items until more is known. Yes, they are popular, have been around for a while, and make cleaning up a lot faster and easier. However, there may be tradeoffs to convenience.

Pumpkin-Cheese Pie

(Smooth, bland)
Makes 8 Servings

8-inch, ready-to-fill graham cracker pie shell, or use Gingersnap Pie
    Shell (see recipe)
1 cup cooked or canned plain pumpkin
3 eggs or the equivalent in egg substitute
1 tbsp artifical rum flavoring or vanilla extract
pinch of salt
1/4 cup brown sugar
1 1/2 cups low-fat creamed cottage cheese
1 1/2 pumpkin pie spices or your preference of nutmeg, cinnamon,
    and allspice

Preheat oven to 275°F before beginning preparation. Combine all ingredients (except pie shell, of course) in a blender and blend on high speed until very smooth. Pour into pie shell and bake for 1 hour or more, until filling is set. Chill before serving.

Beverages

Charger

(Bitter)

Makes 1 serving

Add 2 dashes Angostura bitters and lime wedge to a tall glass. Add sparkling water and ice.

Banana-Peanut Power Shake

(Earthy)

Makes 1 (8-oz) serving

4 oz honey-vanilla yogurt

2 tbsp peanut butter

1 ripe banana

3 tbsp nonfat dry milk or protein soy powder

6 small ice cubes, or 4 large ones

Place ingredients in blender in order listed. Blend until all ice is crushed. (I know that most blender manufacturers say never put ice in a blender, but I've been using ice in my blender for years and it's still whirring away.) Serve immediately.

Barley Tea

(Hot, bland)

1/4 cup organic pearl barley

8 cups of water

If you have an old crock pot sitting around, now is the time to get it out. This recipe takes about 1 1/2 hour to make but can easily make itself overnight in a crock pot.

Put the barley in a strainer and rinse. Put water and barley in the crock pot and let simmer until it is reduced to 4 cups of beverage. Strain and drink hot or cold. You can also add a tablespoon of lemon or lime.

One reason to try various teas and beverages is because women with morning sickness, and especially those with hyperemesis, may not be able to drink plain water. Keeping well-hydrated is very important. In caring for thousands of women over many years, water adversity is a hallmark problem associated with nausea. It could be the background taste or smell of water that is repulsive, because pregnant women have altered senses. No one has studied this phenomena, so I'm putting forward my best speculations here. When you add the smallest ingredients to water, it takes on a whole new personality. Consider that there are hardly any calories in Digestive Tea, but there are powerful substances contributed by spices. In Barley Tea, there are a few calories from carbohydrates and some flavoring from the citrus juices.

Digestive Tea

(Hot, spicy, earthy)

2 cups of water
1 tsp each of coriander seeds, fennel seeds, and cumin seeds.

Boil the water. Put all the seeds in a blender and pour in the boiling water and blend for 15 seconds. Strain the tea into another container. Drink after any meal, hot or cold, depending on your preference.

Homemade Ginger Ale

(Spicy)

Makes 4 (10-oz) servings

This recipe is another used with the permission of Nancy Clark, R.D., M.S., author of *Nancy Clark's Sports Nutrition Cookbook* and other great books on nutrition.

In many eastern countries, ginger has been touted for years as a natural antinauseant, which may explain why some women with nausea gravitate to the more tart and tangy ginger ales. But authorities are quick to point out that there is a difference between fresh and dried gingers, and between ginger from western countries and that from eastern countries. If you find ginger helpful, try ginger conserves on your morning toast.

2 tbsp fresh ginger root, chopped

Rinds of 2 lemons

3–4 tbsp honey or other sweetener to taste

1 cup boiling water

1 quart seltzer (cold)

Put ginger and lemon rinds in a small bowl with honey. Pour in 1 cup boiling water (or just enough to cover). Let steep for 5 minutes. Strain and chill. When ready to serve, add chilled seltzer.

Hot Nutmeg and Ginger Milk

(Spicy, hot)

8 oz low-fat milk

1/2 tsp freshly grated nutmeg if you have it, or powdered baking nutmeg

1/2 tsp grated fresh ginger

Add honey to taste

One of my favorite cookbooks is Christine McFadden's *A Harvest of Healing Foods: Recipes and Remedies for the Mind, Body, and Soul.* The title already suggests you are on your way to feeling better! It provides nutrient breakdown of all the recipes and a list of health organizations, such as American Association of Ayurvedic Medicine. (See Chapter 14 for more information about Ayurvedic medicine.) The preparation of this recipe has been streamlined and inspired from Christine's original, and is based on Ayurvedic principles.

In a 12-ounce coffee mug, pour in 8 ounces of low-fat milk and microwave on medium about 1 minute. You'll need to watch the microwave so you don't boil it over. (The mug will be very hot, so be careful not to burn yourself.) Stir in the nutmeg, ginger, and honey and put back into the microwave to reheat for about 15 seconds. Strain the mixture into another coffee mug and sip.

If you don't have fresh ginger, use 1 tsp of ginger jam and forget the honey. Feel free to vary the amount of ginger and nutmeg to suit your palate.

Indian Yogurt Drink (Lassi)

(Wet)

Makes 4 (1-cup) servings

8 oz plain yogurt

2 pints water

Ice cubes

1 tsp dried mint

1 tsp salt

Mix yogurt and water in large pitcher. Add mint and salt and mix well. Add ice cubes and serve. You can make a large portion of this and freeze it.

Mixed Fruity Shake

(Tangy)
Makes 4 servings

1 1/4 cup cleaned fresh berries or frozen (blueberries, blackberries or strawberries)
1 large banana
2 cups skim milk buttermilk
2–5 tbsp sugar
1/2 tsp grated lemon rind from fresh lemon

Put fruit, buttermilk and sugar in blender and blend for 30 seconds. Add lemon rind, lemon juice and blend 5 seconds. Serve as frappe or make into frozen Popsicle.

Rice Water

(Bland, cold)
Makes 2–3 servings

1 tbsp rice
2 cups cold water or milk
1 tsp sugar
Add cinnamon, nutmeg, or orange or lemon peel for flavoring

Put rice into a pan with water or milk and cook over moderate heat. Bring to boil and then simmer for 30 minutes. Strain and add sugar, spice, or orange or lemon peel as you want. (Or allow rice to cool and blend it and liquid in blender for added calories and thickness.) Chill and serve.

TOPPINGS

Miriam's Ginger-Honey

(Sweet, tangy)
Makes 8 servings

1/2 cup wild honey
1 tsp minced ginger root

Put honey and ginger in a ceramic coffee cup and heat in microwave for 1 minute. This helps develop the flavor. Cover and refrigerate. Use in 1 week. Add to tea, pancakes, or toast.

Miriam's Ginger-Maple Syrup

(Earthy, spicy)
Makes 8 servings

1/2 cup pure maple syrup
1 tsp minced ginger root

Put maple syrup and ginger in a ceramic coffee cup and heat in microwave for 1 minute. Cover and refrigerate. Use in a week. Add to tea, pancakes, or plain cooked white rice with milk for a breakfast food.

OTHER PRODUCTS TO TRY

As a culinary pioneer, it's important to find new food solutions for morning-sickness moms. But the motto is taste before you suggest—especially to a queasy person. Tastes are hard to describe to a well person, and harder yet for a queasy soul.

Here's a list of a few things I've sampled recently. Don't spend huge amounts of money buying tons before you see if one sample has any value to you. There's no conflict of interest on my part with these items; I don't own any stock.

Tazo: Nice, earthy label design with the promise of being the "reincarnation tea." They have a Lemon Ginger iced tea, which is an iced herbal tea with ginger juice and ginseng. It's caffeine free. In 14 ounces, you'll get 70 calories, 17 grams in sugar. Don't expect any vitamins and minerals here. In Boston, I found this tea in a mega grocery store. If it works to calm a queasy stomach, go for it. I don't believe the amount of ginseng in here is a worry.

Glaceau Vitamin Water: I like the one with the name "Rescue" on it! It has a green band on the label to distinguish it from their other products. I found this in Trader Joe's. It contains rosemary, chamomile, hibiscus, lavender, rosehips, and some other herbs. This product does contain 100 percent of the RDI for vitamin C (for nonpregnant people), which is important, and a few B vitamins. You'll get about 125 calories in the 20-oz bottle. It has a pleasant aroma.

enhance: This is an energy formula with taurine and electrolytes. I tried the lemon-lime flavor. The 16-oz bottle has 200 percent of the RDI for vitamin C, a little potassium, and some vitamin B_6. If the flavor is something that works for you, great. Many fruit juices will contain more potassium and vitamin C than glitzy fluids, but sometimes trying something new is helpful.

Dutch Ginger Loaf from JB Bussink: Also in Trader Joe's I found this low-fat ginger loaf. It's about the size of a brick, and it weighs about as much as brick too! It's very dense, but it's a wheat-free and egg-free product for women who have food allergies. You can eat it plain. Try it as a gingerbread pudding (see the recipe for Miriam's Gluten-Free Gingerbread Pudding). It's really tasty—if you like ginger.

Other ginger food products to try include ginger conserve on toast, crystallized baker's ginger pieces, Reed's Jamaican Ginger Beer. It's not real beer; it's a super-duper ginger ale that seems to have more nausea-reducing power.

Another of the quasi-nutritional items to try are the Preggie Pops. The glorified lollipops come in various flavors of mint, ginger, and lavender. The main ingredient is sugar and corn syrup and coloring is added from red cabbage, tumeric, annatto and beet color. Expect to pay about a few dollars for one. That's rather hefty price for 60 calories, but if they work for you, they're worth it. For more information, www.preggiepops.com, or call them at 1-866-PREGGIE. That's a toll-free, 24-hour number.

Cinnamon products work too. Try a red fire ball. They also travel under the name of Atomic Fireballs, I believe.

Chapter 13

Alternative Therapies: Acupuncture

LORI

Although 50 to 90 percent of pregnant women have some degree of morning sickness, Lori found that she had a dreadful case and nothing in the traditional line of fire worked for her. She, being a savvy dietitian, had tried everything under the sun. Finally, she engaged the services of an acupuncturist, who had been a labor and delivery nurse before training to become acupuncturist. Lori wrote that the relief after acupuncture was wonderful, and she started to feel better after week 16. However, every now and then, Lori would test the limits of this therapy. When she would discontinue treatment for over 4 or 5 days, she'd regret it, because she'd suffer a relapse. She also tried ginger products, but they did not work for her. The explanation given by her nurse-acupuncturist was that she had too much internal heat, and ginger, being a warming herb, was contraindicated in this situation.

ACUPUNCTURE AND MORNING SICKNESS

Not surprising, research indicates that women suffering from morning sickness are concerned about the potential adverse effects of prescription medication on fetal development and often consider other noninvasive therapies. This has piqued investigation into alternatives remedies—from devices (sea bands), supplements (vitamin B_6, pregnancy teas), smell and odor control, massage therapy, and Traditional Chinese Medicine (TCM), notably acupuncture.

Chemotherapy-related nausea and vomiting is said to be reduced by acupuncture and has driven support for acupuncture in morning sickness. A colleague and I conducted a reader survey with *Fit Pregnancy* (SHAPE magazine) about morning sickness and found that only 12 of 122 women (9.8 percent) reported using acupuncture. Only 16.7 percent (i.e., 2 of the 12 women) reported an efficacy rating of 60 to 80 percent with acupuncture. The survey, however, failed to account for the various acupoints that may be used, so no information was obtained on which of the many points these two women used. And as we know, there are many variables that affect morning-sickness severity.

ACUPUNCTURE BASICS

Acupuncture, an ancient therapy, is approximately 3,000 years old. It is a highly complex component of Chinese medicine, and the operating principles are based upon meridians. The human body has 12 meridians, also called Ching. Meridians are a concept in Chinese medicine that relate to channels of energy—Chi or Qi, considered the life force—through which energy is channeled that directs the function of various body organs. According to Dr. Kuen-Shii Tsay, professor in the Department of Traditional Chinese Medicine at the New England School of Acupuncture in Watertown, Massachusetts, when Chi flows optimally, we are healthy. When Chi is slow or stuck, we are out of sorts. Dr. Tsay has practiced acupuncture for dozens of years and also is an author of one of the most respected books on the topic, *The Acupuncturist's Handbook: A Practical Encyclopedia*. To realign Chi, needles are placed strategically on the body to correct the imbalance. The points at which needles are inserted are called acupoints. These acupoints are placed on the body according to body maps that are thousands of years old.

In addition, there are eight channels or Ch'i Ching Mei (described as being outside the meridians) and conjunctive channels called Le Mei. Meridians are designated either Yin or Yang (which are known as energy flows) and infiltrate various organs, as noted in Table 13.1. According to practitioners of acupuncture, syndromes of Zang-Fu (meaning the internal organs) are covered by manipulating various acupoints of such organs.

Abbreviations for various acupoints have been standardized for ease of use and accuracy for acupuncturists and are a form of shorthand that has been universally agreed upon. For example, CO stands for colon, which is the large intestine, and LU means lungs.

Table 13.1

Yang	Yin
Large intestine (CO)	Lungs (LU)
Stomach (ST)	Spleen (SP)
Small intestine (SI)	Heart (HE)
Tri-heaters (TH)	Heart-constrictors (HC)
Gallbladder (GB)	Liver (LI)

GB-14 stands for gallbladder, and the number 14 indicates that it is the 14th acupuncture point on the gallbladder meridian. You can imagine that the possibilities for needle placement are pretty vast.

There were originally 365 acupuncture points, corresponding precisely with the number of days in the year. Reportedly, it expanded to as many as 1,000 needling sites over time, however, fewer than 100 points are commonly used by practitioners today. You might also hear about other aspects of acupuncture, for example, electric acupuncture and moxibustion. Moxibustion is the application of heat to acupuncture points by burning moxa (also known as *ai* in TCM), the dried leaves of *Artemisia vulgaris* (mugwort). Moxa can be used alone or as a complement to acupuncture.

Within this complex system are major meridians that can be used:

Lung meridian of hand
Large intestine meridian of hand
Stomach meridian of foot
Spleen meridian of foot
Heart meridian of hand
Small intestine meridian of hand
Urinary bladder meridian of foot
Kidney meridian of foot
Pericardium meridian of hand
Triple warmer meridian of hand
Gallbladder meridian of foot
Liver meridian of foot
Conception vessel meridian
Governor vessel meridian

You might be getting an idea of just how complicated successful acupuncture can be!

RESEARCH ON ACUPUNCTURE

Given the various points used in pregnancy, at least two researchers tried to see which combination seemed to produce the best results. A group from Exeter, England, conducted a randomized, controlled trial of acupuncture for morning sickness. Fifty-five women with nausea, with or without vomiting, were randomly assigned to the acupuncture or placebo (toothpicks) group as outpatients. It is hard to know what level of nausea the study subjects had on the beginning day of therapy. The symptoms the women reported during the prior week were the determining factors for the group to which they were assigned, and all reported moderate to severe nausea in the previous week. All women were between 6 to 10 weeks pregnant and were an average age of 30 years old. In the acupuncture group, 14 women were first-time moms and 14 already had at least one child. The women were an average weight of 138 pounds, or 62.8 kilograms. In the toothpick group of 27, 9 were first-time moms and 18 already had at least one baby. The average weight for this group was heavier by about 13 pounds, or 6 kilograms—a difference of 9 percent. Each group received self-help lists for rest and food choices.

At the first visit for care, each woman was given one of three acupuncture treatments and assigned to group 1, 2, or 3 based on various characteristics. Remember, some women received real needles, and some received toothpicks held in place.

Group 1: Stomach and spleen *qi xu*, or conception vessel (CV) 6, for nausea, stuffiness in the chest, and lassitude, with pale white, moist tongue, and slippery (or weak) pulse. CV 6 refers to a location on the abdomen, below the navel. Presumably, the acupuncturist stimulates this point where there are disorders associated with the kidney or irregular menstruation. For women with these symptoms, the following acupuncture points were used:

Stomach 36 (below the knee)
Conception 12 (central upper abdomen)
Spleen 4 (medial border of the foot, right side only)
Pericardium 6 (medial surface of the wrist)

The numbers associated with the locations, such as stomach 36, are terms that have been translated from the original Chinese description. These abbreviations are universal because Chinese is a difficult language for nonnative speakers to learn.

Group 2: Stomach fire; for lump in throat; heartburn; metal taste in mouth; constant hunger; sour regurgitation; constipation; nausea and vomiting immediately after eating; red tongue with yellow, cracked coat; and rapid, slippery, full pulse. (Stomach fire is a complicated acupuncture term that is almost synonymous with heartburn. It is described as burning pain in the stomach region accompanied by vomiting, a bitter taste in the mouth, foul breath, swollen gums, constipation, an irregular and rapid pulse, and a rough, red tongue with a yellow coating.) These women were given acupuncture using the following points:

Stomach 44 (forefoot)
Conception vessel 12
Pericardium 6

Group 3: Heat in heart and disharmony of liver, for nausea, bitter taste, restlessness, insomnia, vivid dreams, thirst, dark urine, red tongue with red spots on tip and yellow coat, and rapid, slippery, wiry pulse. (*Disharmony of the liver* refers to the constellation of symptoms of nausea, vomiting, and abdominal pain. When a liver is diseased, Western medicine would refer to this as abnormal liver function, whereas Eastern medicine would refer to it as disharmony of the liver.) Acupuncture points were different for this group and included:

Conception vessel 12
Stomach 34
Pericardium 6

Whether the women received toothpicks or needles, each was left in position 15 minutes. All women were treated twice in the first week, once in the second week, and once in the third week. Most reduction in nausea occurred within the first 2 days. A few adverse reactions were noted in the needle group: two cases of tiredness, sleep disturbance, heaviness of arms, bruising, pressure in the nose, and headache. In the toothpick group, there were two cases of tiredness and altered taste, one case each of increased vomiting, intestinal gas, vivid dreams, and feelings of coldness. All women were evaluated for anxiety and depression. The researchers observed that the women in the toothpick group had somewhat more anxiety and depression, but no severe emotional problems were noted. The toothpick group was heavier overall, but there is no way to know for sure whether that made any difference.

Both groups had a reduction in nausea! Nausea scores decreased from 85.5 to 47.5 in the needle group and from 87.0 to 48.0 in the toothpick group. The researchers believed nausea reduction was the result of stimulating A-delta nerve fibers in skin and muscle. Four treatment sessions were given over 3 weeks. Both groups of women were reported to be pleased to talk about their morning-sickness therapies.

There did not appear to be a huge difference in symptom relief between the toothpick group and needle group, and women in both groups reported improvement. In acupuncture, needles are inserted to elicit a *Deqi* sensation. Deqi is described as a dull aching sensation that is believed to be associated with the correct position of the needle. The type of treatment given to the needle group would be considered deep needling, whereas the toothpick treatment would be considered light manipulation and did not evoke any reported sensations. Before dismissing the claims of improvement in the toothpick group, one might consider that the improvement experienced might have been caused by reduced levels of the stress hormone cortisol as a result of feeling cared for (of course, the same could be said of any treatment in which the patient receives a lot of individual intention). Lying down in a restful position could also have made the difference. What matters is that both groups of women experienced relief.

Whether the difference in weight of 9 percent between the two groups in the Exeter trial would result in a difference of acupuncture effectiveness is not known. A shallower needling depth is recommended for children and slim clients, whereas greater needling depth is recommended for athletic and obese clients. Severe or chronic disease profiles tend to require deeper needling; however, it is not clear where morning sickness or hyperemesis gravidarum fall in terms of depth of tonifying, so be sure to ask your acupuncturist. Angles of inserted needles can also vary from 90 degrees to 30 to 50 or 5 to 15 degrees. Needles may also be rotated (90 or 180 degrees) as well as lifted and depressed to achieve a tonifying effect (4 to 8 Hz or 1 to 2 Hz). Whether the reduction in morning-sickness symptoms from these studies can be based on acupuncture alone is difficult to know. Dietary choices can make a difference.

Another study was carried out in Sweden. Although about 72 women were approached for the study, in the end, only 33 completed the study. Women were hospitalized for 8 days. Group A, with 17 women, underwent deep acupuncture treatments for $2\frac{1}{2}$ days, with a 2-day break and then very light acupuncture treatments from day 4.5 to day 8. Group B, with 16 women, was only lightly acupunctured. All women received sugar or glucose water. Both deep and light acupuncture treatments used the pericardium 6 (PC 6, or Neiguan in Chinese) point, which is located on the wrist. These treatments were given three times daily on treatment days for 30 minutes. The Deqi sensation meant the needles were inserted deeply enough, and were twisted according to tradition. In the light acupuncture group, no Deqi sensations were searched out, but the needles were twisted a little every 10 minutes of treatment.

Both groups of women needed less intravenous fluids after admission. There were no adverse side effects during or after the study. Women were allowed to eat, but we don't know what they actually did consume. The analysis showed a significant and faster reduction of nausea when women received the real therapy rather than the light therapy.

Two studies from China show some differences in treatment but positive outcomes. Zhao Rongun treated 39 cases of morning sickness with acupuncture. Again, depending on which of the three traditional diagnoses of morning sickness variety was made— stomach-deficiency type, liver-heat type, and phlegm-damp type— the acupuncture sites differed. Main acupuncture points used for the stomach-deficiency types were bilateral Zusanli (ST 36) and bilateral Taichong (LI 3) with auxiliary points of Zhongwan (Ren 12) and Neiguan (PC 6). (*Bilateral* means that two needles were used and placed at even distance from the acupuncture location. If a third location is used, it is called an *auxiliary* point.)

Again, in Chinese medicine, the description of a person's illness will determine which acupoints are used. Some morning-sickness women are described in acupuncture terms as having more trouble with their stomachs (probably intense and unremitting nausea); some might have more liver problems (probably losing weight, vomiting green bile, and heading to gallbladder disease); and some have bigger complaints of saliva or phlegm (probably ptylism gravidarum, the incessant pregnancy drool).

Main points used for the liver-heat type were bilateral Taichong (LI 3) and bilateral Zusanli (ST 36) with an auxiliary point of Yanglingquan (GB 34).

The phlegm-damp types were treated with main points of bilateral Fenglong (ST 40) and bilateral Zusanli (ST 36) with an auxiliary point of Neiguan (PC 6). Needles were in place for 30 to 40 minutes, during which time they were manipulated 2 to 3 times. Treatment was twice daily at 6 to 8 hour intervals, then once a day after improvement was noted. In six cases, acupuncture proved effective after 2 days of treatment. In 31 cases it was effective after 3 to 5 days. In one case it was effective after 5 days. Overall effectiveness was 97 percent.

In the second paper I reviewed by Zhao Changxin, moxa was also added. Again, the morning-sickness groups were described in terms of stomach deficiency, liver heat, and stagnancy of phlegm as well as by acupuncture points.

For stomach deficiency, points used were Zhongwan (Ren 12), Zusanli (ST 36), and Gongsun (SP 4). Mild moxibustion or moxiacupuncture could be used. For liver-heat types, the points used were Taichong (LI 3), Yinlingquan (GB 24), Zhongwan (Ren 12), and Zusanli (ST 36). For stagnancy of phlegm, points used were Fenglong (ST 40), Yinlingquan (GB 24), Zusanli (ST 36), and Zhongwan (Ren 12).

Ear acupuncture therapy can also be used. You can stimulate points for the stomach, liver, and spleen—up to 20 minutes a day on each ear. In all categories, it is suggested to treat once a day, retaining needles for 20 minutes. If necessary, treat twice a day.

Looking through a few acupuncture books, I noticed other points offered. It's certainly not a case of one size fits all! You should keep track of your type of morning sickness and the acupoints used by providers. A chart is provided at the end of this chapter to help you organize information about your acupuncture treatment. Being able to compare your data with that of other women would certainly be helpful.

DURATION OF RELIEF

The Swedish research group found that relief lasts approximately eight hours, which prompted administration of acupuncture three times a day in their study. Presumably, acupuncture analgesia achieves its maximum level within 20 to 30 minutes, has a half-life of 15 to 17 minutes upon removal of the needles, exhibits a slow onset, and wears off slowly.

SAFETY OF ACUPUNCTURE

One investigator found that practitioners observed one adverse event for every 8 to 9 months of full-time practice or one adverse event for every 633 consultations. Adverse reactions reported include local and systemic infections, such as endocarditis, septicemia, hepatitis B, human immunodeficiency virus (HIV) infection, osteomyelitis, myositis, peritonitis, and pleural empyema.

When choosing an acupuncturist, you'll need to pay attention to the titles acupuncturists use, because they are not standard. It seems that some of the states that offer the most prestigious licensure titles do not always require the highest educational standards. Talk with your obstetrician before you begin acupuncture therapy (or any therapy for that matter) to reduce morning sickness. Seek out a certified acupuncturist if you want to learn more about acupuncture.

HOW DOES ACUPUNCTURE WORK?

In 1997 the National Institutes of Health (NIH) held a 3-day conference on acupuncture. Unfortunately, the conference did not address using acupuncture on pregnant women. Most comments about acupuncture and nausea and vomiting were from work done on postoperative (surgery) and chemotherapy patients.

Research in acupuncture (especially electroacupuncture) for pain management indicates that the brain has developed complex systems for diminishing or enhancing pain perception. As you'd expect, the brain is highly complex. There are approximately 50 different neurotransmitters (brain chemicals) identified in the human brain that are affected by acupuncture.

According to presentations at NIH, acupuncture has been shown to reduce pain perception by increasing pain threshold, ease symptoms of depression, increase gastric motility, improve immune function, induce ovulation in certain situations, and reduce blood fat levels.

Acupuncture's success on reducing pain perception is an important consideration. One researcher at Stanford University found a common dopaminergic receptor gene that tied adverse smells, bad morning sickness, and migraine headaches together. This finding gave researchers more information about how the brain functions. Many women with morning sickness also complain about headaches, not necessarily migraine headaches. Acupuncture has been reported to be helpful in alleviating headaches. Dr. Heinrich compared the agony of hyperemesis to delivery and said that "the majority of women reported that the pain experienced during vomiting exceeded that of parturition [delivery]." Dr. Heinrich is part of the obstetrical department at Stanford, so he's seen a lot of women with this problem.

OTHER CONSIDERATIONS FOR ACUPUNCTURE TREATMENT

Acupuncture for morning sickness may well work for some women and should be considered. Check to see whether your insurance will cover the cost of a visit and how far you have to drive for an appointment. You should review the potential risks with the provider, and get his or her track record for success with morning-sickness clients. If a referral is made for acupuncture, you'll need to be informed of the potential risk, the limited duration of relief, that multiple acupoints may be used, and that you may experience side effects. You'll want to discuss the use of moxa, as well as many other herbs that might be suggested, with your obstetrician.

I'd suggest that anyone who uses acupuncture for morning sickness keep a diary of acupoints used during treatment, diet, weather, and all those other variables we've discussed. You might spot a pattern in what aggravates or alleviates your symptoms.

Use this chart when you are calling acupuncturists. Share the information with your obstetrician.

Acupuncturist name:_____

Address: _____

Phone number:_____

Number of morning-sickness women treated: _____

Success level:_____

School trained: _____

Specialties:_____

Credentials: _____

My Traditional Chinese morning-sickness type is_____, based on_____.

Acupoints: _____

Rating therapy: Day 1   Day 2   Day 3

_____

Other thoughts:_____

_____

Week of pregnancy and other therapies used:_____

_____

If you think the concept of acupuncture is worth a trial but are afraid of needles, consider reading *Acupuncture without Needles*, by J.V. Cherney. This book is described as do-it-yourself acupressure—the simple, at-home treatment for lasting relief from pain. It is very user-friendly and has a great diagram of acupoints on the bottom of the feet to consider as well as dozens of diagrams of pressure points throughout the body.

Another therapy to consider is a variation of acupressure: reflexology. Reflexology uses acupoints in the hands and feet to try to correct the body's disharmony. A reference I would suggest is Rosalind Oxenford's book *Instant Reflexology for Stress Relief: Simple Techniques to Relieve Stress and Enhance Your Mind*. It has a great foot chart that depicts points that should be pressed. Reflexology might be just the thing to get you some relief—a foot massage is generally pleasant. I recall one woman I cared for in two horrific pregnancies who reported that the only relief she got was when her husband massaged her feet. He had an innate ability to know just where to massage. For partners who aren't that naturally gifted, Oxenford's book is reasonably priced and might be worth its weight in gold.

LORI'S ACUPUNCTURIST

Thanks to the Internet, I was able to ask Lori's acupuncturist, Liz Walters, about her track record. Liz is a registered nurse who trained as an acupuncturist. She operates Dancing Cranes. She has treated several women who had hyperemesis. Everyone got relief for at least 3 days. Two women came weekly until they hit the second trimester. Some women stopped therapy because of work schedules or money issues. She doesn't use the same therapy on everyone. Like you've read earlier, the traditional Chinese system recognizes more than one diagnosis for morning sickness. If you live in the northwest, you might give Liz a call. Or e-mail her at liz@dancingcranes.net.

Chapter 14

Alternative Remedies: Other Things Women Try

ALMAZ

The list of suggestions was endless for Almaz, the 15-year-old immigrant from Somalia. She was suffering badly from morning sickness, and everyone in her community and at the clinic wanted to help. On top of feeling horrible, she was struggling to learn enough English to communicate when her 27-year-old graduate-student husband was unable to accompany her to the local clinic. In a foreign tongue, she could not even begin to adequately articulate just how poorly she was feeling. After her first intake session at the clinic, the interpreter and social worker gave her a picture board with faces—miserable to happy—to use for a quick reference.

Almaz, cloaked in her burqa, would often be found on a park bench a few blocks from their student accommodations, incapacitated by nausea. Often one of her neighbors would need to accompany her for the rest of the journey to a local health clinic for fluids. To those who cared for her, she was a bright-eyed girl having her first baby, far from home and suffering from horrible emesis.

Almaz became the girl everyone tried to help at the clinic. Books on herbs were a frequent gift. Someone brought her Sea Bands and electronic Relief Bands. Ginger of all sorts, shapes, and sizes—supplements and food—made their way into the pockets of her caregivers. Most of the time, Almaz was at the clinic long before her scheduled appointments because her morning sickness was so out of control. Vitamin B_6 was suggested, and various homeopathic compounds as well. One provider had spent time reading and investigating medical hypnosis, but Almaz declined. She was not sure how her religious beliefs would mesh with that. Massage was another suggestion, but she dismissed it immediately because of personal modesty issues.

Of all the remedies that were offered, in the end Almaz felt most comfortable with the herbal options. She felt her relatives in Somalia would have done the same. The rest were too foreign to her. Almaz was caught in a cultural and medical divide—the first person of her family in a sophisticated metropolis, where few people understood the best way to treat her.

There was one more thing to be concerned about with Almaz. Being covered up from head to toe reduced her exposure to sunlight. It was therefore important to be sure she had a diet adequate in calcium and vitamin D because she could be at risk for deficiencies. In addition, the vitamin D content of her breast milk could be affected.

FRANCINE

Dubbed "Mrs. Lemonade and potato chips" by her father, Francine was hospitalized on four separate occasions and spent a total of

30 days in the hospital. During the fourth stay, of 19 days, her diet consisted mainly of lemonade frappes and potato chips, both of which were roundly criticized by her family. Up to this time, Frannie said, her coworkers had thought she was just "putting it on" when she complained of nausea and vomiting. Her weight had dropped 20 pounds in 12 weeks, and she was no longer able to function at home or in her office. She had a difficult time walking. She felt she couldn't have been more depressed. "Nothing is fun anymore. Pregnancy is about as much fun as chemotherapy," she thought, "but the chemo patients get some understanding and compassion." When she was asked if she wanted to see the chaplain, she thought. "Can't hurt—unless, of course, he or she wears perfume or cologne and drinks coffee in my room!"

She was visited by an energetic clergy intern whose sister had had hyperemesis. Her clergy counselor knew more about bad morning sickness than she had expected. The clergy intern was able to explain some of the nuances of the waxing and waning course she was going through, and help her find passages in the Bible and in various prayer sources to get her through some of the very dark days.

During one hospital admission, her doctor, an avid sailor, saw an ad in a boating magazine about antiseasickness wristbands. He gave Frannie the clipping, saying that it was worth a gamble. Frannie ordered a set and had them delivered at once. A bead on the band was supposed to exert pressure on a nerve, which, according to the brochure, was connected to the vomiting center in the brain. The speculation was that the pressure controlled the urge to vomit.

In two days she felt better than she had in weeks. She said she felt foolish wearing the scratchy gray elastic bands on her wrists, but, for whatever reason, she made progress. After maintaining stability for two days, she was ready for discharge. As she was walking the long corridors of the hospital, she spied another woman who looked almost as green as she had, with a funky looking device on her wrist, and she wondered its purpose. The two women seemed to know they were the current pukers and stopped to compare notes. What Frannie learned was that Lucy, her newfound kindred spirit, was sporting the newest gadget in emesis management—Relief Bands. Lucy was not convinced that they worked well for her; she had super-hyperemesis, which was more than Relief Bands were designed to handle. Nonetheless, she said the zapping she felt on her wrist at least distracted her enough that she didn't dwell on her stomach.

Meanwhile, Frannie's mother knew discharge was about to happen (again), so she dutifully went off to clean the young couple's apartment. When Frannie entered the spotless rooms and smelled the cleaning agents, she immediately felt nauseated again. She opened a window and stuck her head out for fresh air. She barked at her husband to remove all the pails and bottles of cleaning materials immediately. She told me, "I know my mother didn't understand—she was only trying to help—but the smells were really getting to me. I knew if I started vomiting, I'd be right back in the hospital. And that's about the *last* place you want to be these days! They really start giving you the heave ho—no pun intended—when they see you coming back!"

Francine's relatives bet that the baby would be a girl with lots of hair. According to an old wives' tale, the hair of the unborn fetus aggravates the mother's gastrointestinal tract and causes vomiting. Frannie's husband's family had heard that morning sickness was the result of the double-estrogen theory—the notion that a baby girl's own estrogen is what makes the mother sick.

During her months of waiting, Frannie was able to return to work part-time. She said that she had to open the bus windows in the dead of winter to get gulps of fresh air. Once an older man tried to close the window, and she said simply, "I have really bad morning sickness, and I'm trying not to get sick." He apologized and moved his seat. She also found that when she rode on the bus she had to look straight ahead because sitting sideways made her instantly queasy. Once, on the subway, she felt that too many people were jammed in and "robbed [her] of [her] air." She leaped out at the next stop, seconds before vomiting into a trash can, and peeled off her jacket and scarf, perspiring despite the cold.

Finally, the time came when they became proud parents of a baby boy. Frannie, who admits that she wondered many times while she was vomiting and retching with morning sickness, "Why did I ever want to be pregnant?" now says, "My baby is so wonderful, cheerful, happy. . . . I guess the end had to turn out good because the beginning and the middle were just so horrible." To this day, the reason for the success of the lemonade frappes and potato chips remains a mystery. She wonders if it was the Relief Bands or the medical benefit of spirituality she was learning to practice that made the big difference. Or, it might have been just the tincture of time.

HELP FROM DEVICES AND TECHNIQUES

SEA BANDS

One study from Italy showed that 60 percent of women did better with the elastic Sea Band that had the bead sewn than the women in than the placebo group did with their substitute. These items, generally found in marine shops, are now more common in larger pharmacy chains. They aren't overly expensive, so a trial is suggested. But call to see whether the pharmacy has them in stock before you go out running around to buy them.

Relief Bands

The Relief Band, an electronic zapper, has been shown in studies to help women with mild morning sickness. This gizmo looks like a big Swatch watch, put on to face the inside of the wrist. It emits pulses to the wrist. I tried one of these things at an obstetricians' conference and freaked out a bit. I wasn't expecting to receive mild electric shocks. The sensation wasn't unpleasant, once I knew what to expect. These are not inexpensive, but if they work, the expense would be worth it. There are two models: disposable and rechargeable. If you get one, I'd suggest the rechargeable. See (www.reliefband.com) for more information. Once you are done with it, you could donate it to a cancer care center. If it works to control your nausea, it should help someone with cancer-related nausea. You might be able to deduct the expense from your taxes if you get a receipt for making a charitable donation. Or you could offer it to another woman with hyperemesis.

However, if these things don't seem to work for you, and you keep loosing weight, ask for help and explore another alternative. Nothing works for everyone, and you are not wedded to something that is a failure.

Medical Hypnotherapy or Hypnosis

Some women have misgivings about hypnotherapy, which is often used as a last resort. Dr. Eric Simon, a psychologist in California, says there are several myths that need to be dispelled about this benign therapy. Hypnosis is really a form of self-hypnosis; it does not take control away from a woman. Rather, it can increase one's self-control over physiologic processes. It is not the same as stage hypnosis, where candidates act out of control. It's not a black hole, and it's not a state of sleep. Positive words are repeated by the facilitator to help a woman control breathing, reinforce images of calmness, and relax muscles that can decrease sympathetic nervous system arousal.

FOOT REFLEXOLOGY

There are pressure points on the bottom of the feet that presumably correspond to meridians that induce relaxation. I've seen cute socks with directions to "push here" or "press there" imprinted on them. Since a good foot massage is restful, I'd suggest you investigate this. Some pregnant women report that a foot massage brought them some relief from their nausea. Plus, someone working on your feet doesn't have to worry about breathing pepperoni breathe on you!

I'm sure there are several vendors for these reflexology socks. The socks I'm familiar with, from my local Whole Foods Market, are from Earth Therapeutics (www.earththerapeutics.com). There are books on reflexology that your significant other could check out for you at the library. A good short massage is great, but a long, bad one does absolutely nothing.

HERBAL PREPARATIONS FROM EAST TO WEST

LEARNING ABOUT HERBAL PRODUCTS

There are many references that describe plants, roots, bark, and leaves that have been used to treat nausea and vomiting. However, it's hard to say how efficacious these remedies are because Western medicine does not utilize them regularly. Of course, with all herbs, there are concerns: Pesticide and herbicide use, proper plant identification, active ingredients, processing, and issues of mold contamination, strength of final preparation, dosage to use, and duration of therapy are all very important aspects, in addition to cross-reactivity with any standard Western medicines. If you are considering taking any plant products, working with your registered herbalist and doctor is key. In addition, you can find out information about herbal products from any of the 10 sites around the country who have grants and contracts with the National Institutes of Health (NIH), Complementary and Alternative Medicine divisions. (For more information, visit the NIH Web site: http://www.ccam.nih.gov.) Table 14.1 is a list of the current sites and the area of interest for each of those sites.

Table 14.1 Areas of Research for Current Sites Associated with NIH

Site	Research Focus
Bastyr University at Kenmore, Washington	HIV/AIDS
Columbia University at New York City	Women's health issues
Harvard Medical School, Beth Israel Deaconess Medical Center	General medical conditions
Kessler Institute for Rehabilitation at West Orange, New Jersey	Stroke and neurological conditions
Palmer Center for Chiropractic Research at Davenport, Iowa	Chiropractic
Stanford University at Palo Alto, California	Aging
University of Arizona Health Science Center at Tucson	Pediatric conditions
University of California at Davis	Asthma, allergy, and immunology
University of Maryland at Baltimore	Pain
University of Michigan at Ann Arbor	Cardiovascular disease
University of Minnesota at Minneapolis	Addictions
University of Texas Health Science Center at Houston	Cancer
University of Virginia at Charlottesville	Pain

HELPFUL HERBS TO TRY

Pregnant women have relied on Chinese and other eastern herbal remedies as well as on acupuncture in morning-sickness management. A group from Japan, for example, made two herbal preparations into suppository form and tried them out on women with hyperemesis. Some Chinese herbal products are Hange-koboku-to extract granules (HKT) and Bukuryon-in-go-hange-koboku-to (BIH). HKT was the product of choice for women with nausea or vomiting, whereas BIH was used more for reflux or gastritis. All women apparently received fluid support. The method used to evaluate the effectiveness was quite complicated but, in the end, it appeared that these herbal products worked. Whether these herbs have counterparts in the Western botanical world, we don't know.

Coriander, or what is known in the West as cilantro, can be used for nausea. It is part of the parsley family. The seeds as well as leaves have been used. Cassia has been used for nausea and abdominal pain with vomiting. Cassia is also known as Chinese cinnamon. An agent in cassia, cinnamaldehyde, has been found to have sedative and pain-relieving effects on mice. Luo le, the oriental name for basil, belongs to the mint family and has been used in Chinese and Western folk medicine to treat gastrointestinal problems, vomiting, and indigestion.

Pu gong ying—a member of *Taraxacum officinale*—has been used for years in Eastern medicine to treat chronic gastritis and vomiting. You might have a tough time finding any of this fresh, untainted plant in the United States. It's common name is *dandelion!*

Shi luo zi, or xiao hui xiang—known as small fennel—is used as an antispasmodic because it contains carvones, coumarins, bergaptaen, scopoletin, umbelliferones, flavonoids, and phenolic acids, among it's other helpful properties of increasing appetite, treating upset stomach, and decreasing flatulence. You know Shi luo zi as dill.

Shogaols is one of the many ingredients you'll find in sheng jiang—the fresh root—or in gan jiang, it's dried equivalent. It has been used for centuries for nausea and vomiting. Another active ingredient in this plant is gingerols. You guessed it—it's ginger!

The three relatives of the genus *Mentha* are used in Traditional Chinese Medicine (TCM). *Mentha piperita* is peppermint, *Mentha spicata* is spearmint, and *Mentha arvenis* is cornmint. Cornmint, or bo he, is said to have cooling properties and is used extensively in TCM, whereas the other two mints are the opposite, or warming. The use of plants in the genus *Mentha* is complicated because of the assigned properties. Spearmint and peppermint have been used to treat nausea.

Jie Zi (brown mustard seeds) and Bai jie zi (white mustard seeds) have been used in treating vomiting and stomachaches for many centuries. Their botanical families differ. White mustard is thought to have originated in the Mediterranean region, whereas brown mustard is native to Asia. Now both are universally available.

Rou dou kou from the species *Myristica fragrans* is considered a calmative; that is, it settles the stomach. This spice, commonly known as nutmeg, is used in Western folk medicine and in Chinese medicine to treat lack of appetite, reduce vomiting, and stimulate digestion.

Papaya, *Carica papaya*, a tropical fruit known in Oriental medicine as fan mu gua, has been used to treat indigestion and stomachaches. It's a fruit loaded with vitamins and minerals. For folks with super latex allergies, this food, among others, can precipitate a crisis. It's rare, but if you are among the small percentage with severe latex-diet syndrome, you'll want to stay clear of this food in any form whatsoever. This example of potential adversity is why you must never take anything without completely documented knowledge of what's in it. What papaya and latex share in common is a protein or a peptide. If you don't know which foods can cause complications for people who have latex-diet syndrome, see the appendix.

Mei gui hua and qiang wei hua are forms of rose that can be added to food to improve digestion and counter lack of appetite. I found an interesting product at Whole Foods Market—a spritzer bottle of rose water. This is food grade so you can spritz it on something like rice as well as on your body. Rose water is commonly added to foods from India, and you probably never had any idea.

Mi die xiang translates to rosemary, part of the mint family, and it is used by some Eastern cultures to treat stomach pains.

Star anise has a long history in Chinese medicine for therapies of the stomach. It is related to the magnolia family and is called ba jiao hui xiang (small star anise), not to be confused with da hui xiang (meaning large fennel)—both are used in TCM. (Chinese star anise has sometimes been confused with the Japanese star anise.) Japanese star anise has different components, which in large amounts are toxic. The Chinese star anise is often combined with ginger and clove for treating nausea and vomiting.

Suan dour (or suan jiao), meaning sour bean or sour fruit, is a relative of the pea family, but it is actually a large evergreen tree. The ripe or almost ripe fruit is used as a medicine and a food. This is the tamarind, highly recommended to pregnant women for the treatment of morning sickness. It has been identified as having both sweet and sour properties, and it is of a cooling nature. Tamarind pods are sold in ethnic markets, in health food stores, and in some large supermarkets. I've tried dried tamarind—to me it tasted sour and salty.

Thyme, or she xiang cao, has been used as a tea for lack of appetite. The thematic grouping is one way that some herbalists classify herbs. Thyme has been associated with respiratory, digestive, and reproductive health. Thyme is also thought to have some antiseptic properties. The quantity of thyme that would be needed to produce these effects is not known; however, the amount that one enjoys having added to food is determined by the individual palate, which imposes its own restrictions.

"Spices as Medicinal Remedies" is one of the last chapters in *The Indonesian Kitchen*, a fascinating book. They suggest a number of spices for various conditions: cardamom for stomach disturbances; chili for lack of appetite; citrus leaves for fatigue; cloves for stomach disturbances; coriander for stomach disturbances; cumin for stomach disturbances; garlic for migraines; ginger root for poor appetite, digestion, headache, and vomiting; kencur root for vomiting; laos root for stomach disturbances; lemon grass to increase appetite and help prevent vomiting; nutmeg and onions for vomiting; salam leaves for a weak stomach; and tamarind for apathy and nervousness.

You might get the feeling that if you add a few herbs and seasonings to your common diet, maybe there would be a therapeutic result. That's one way that seems to work. Dig through cookbooks from your background as well as from other cultures for recipes that use some of these ingredients. Some culinary experimentation just might prove effective. Remember, however, that cooking smells can contribute to the problem of nausea. Cooking smells are very different during the course of food preparation. It's best to sit down and sample a ready-made meal— made someplace other than in your own home.

Although many herbs have helpful effects, pregnant women should never self-medicate with herbs. Always consult your obstetricians before taking any substance.

AYURVEDIC HEALTH PRACTICES

The practice of Ayurvedics is fascinating. It is the natural traditional healing system of India, a system that combines diet, healing, and health maintance with a deep spiritual commitment to nature. The term Ayurveda is Sanskrit for "the knowledge of life or daily living" and thus emphasizes that humans come from nature, that we are an integral part of the universe, and that we have a responsibility to it—the balance of the universe lives within us all. Personalities are described in three ways: *vata, pitta,* and *kapha.*

The vata personality is described as being on the go all the time; the pitta is blessed with lots of determination and a strong will; and the kapha is endowed with strength, endurance, and stamina. Although these personality traits are pretty general, Ayurevedics also outlines the general traits of each personality that lead to health decline. For the vata, too much worrying, not getting enough rest, and not keeping a routine are typical problems. For the pitta, drinking too much alcohol, eating too many spicy or salty foods, and engaging in too many frustrating activities are hallmarks. The kapha type takes too many naps after meals, eats too many fatty foods, can easily become a couch potato, and luxuriates in inertia. I'm sure we are all a blend of these types from time to time!

Taste, or *rasa,* is a key component of understanding Ayurvedic nutrition. In addition, a food with heat is thought to enhance digestion, whereas a food with cold components is thought to slow it down. The key to good digestion—called digestive fire or agni—

is based on good health and overall strength. Herbs are used extensively in Ayurvedic medicine to stimulate digestion and enhance nutrient absorption. In addition, there are about 10 nutrition principles that include very common-sense reminders. Two of these are that eating should not be rushed and that foods need to be eaten in the proper amounts—not too much or too little. You might want to further explore Ayurveda if you find relief from the Digestive or Barley Tea recipes in Chapter 12, "Recipes and Menus."

HOMEOPATHY

Homeopathy is a complex area of treatment; the information in this section is based on a search of the traditional medical literature, using the keywords of *homeopathy* and *morning sickness*, and *hyperemesis gravidarum*. Any pregnant women considering homeopathic therapies needs to talk to her obstetrician beforehand. Although homeopathy has been used for over 200 years, there are still a lot of unanswered questions about how it works and what it does. The Centers of Complementary and Alternative Medicine branch of the NIH are studying homeopathy, among other medical therapies. However, no center is enrolling pregnant women into studies, so data about efficacy and safety are lacking. To date, European countries have the most experience with using homeopathic therapies.

Homeopathy is based on the principle that, if a lot of something will make you sick, a little of it will make your immune system stronger. Established by German physician Samuel Hahnemann (1755–1843), homeopathy embraces concepts such as the Law of Similars, the Law of Cures, and Provings. In practice, some substances that have been acknowledged to be toxic or poisonous in their crude state are used after dilution with alcohol. Among the substances so used are flowers, leaves, seeds, roots, barks, and resins. Homeopathy also uses degradation products such as petroleum and charcoal, as well as mosses, lichens, and mushrooms.

Mineral remedies are also used, for example, ores, acids, alkalis, and salts. Animal products are also part of the homeopathic bag of tricks and include venoms of jellyfish, insects, spiders, mollusks, crustaceans, fish, amphibians, snakes, and other reptiles. Products of living things are also used: milks, hormones, glandular and tissue extracts, and disease products of nosodes derived from tuberculosis, gonorrhea, abscesses, pathogenic bacteria, and vaccines. (Nosodes essentially translates into the practice of using diseased substances or tissues mixed with alcohol as therapeutic agents. An example of this would be using a respiratory discharge, mixed with alcohol, as a medicine.)

Homeopaths use the least amount of agent possible. Solutions are diluted according to factors of 10. This is a mind-boggling way to try to keep track. For example, 6X, 12X, and 30X are common concentrations you might see on labels. A concentration of 6X means six dilutions of 1:10, or 10 to the minus 6 power; 12X means 12 dilutions of 1:10, or 10 to the minus 12 power. According to Dr. Richard Moskowitz, a homeopathic obstetrician and author of *Homeopathic Medicines for Pregnancy and Childbirth*, this means that 6X is really 1 part in 1 million, or a very dilute solution, especially in the self-care arena.

Some of the suggested homeopathic remedies for morning sickness are nux vomica, which is really strychnine; cocculus, which is powdered Indian cockle, a plant; colchicum, which is the bulb of meadow safron; ipecac, which is made fron the dried rhizome or root of Cephaelis acuminata or Cephaelis ipecacuanha, two tropical American plants; and *Symphoricarpos*, a ripe snowberry. Sepia is also used for those with nausea and vomiting of pregnancy, who are overly sensitive to smells and motion. Sepia is the ink of a cuttlefish, called *Sepia officinalis*.

Two other agents might be recommended: *Magnesia phosphorica* as an antispasmodic and colocynthis, which is the tincture of the fruit pulp of the bitter cucumber, or *Cucumis colocynthis*.

Olive is used to restore energy when you are physically and mentally exhausted. Oak is the presumed cure that the naturally strong should take when they need a break. (I'd say, "take a break!") Willow is supposed to allow you to forgive past injustices and move on when you feel resentful and bitter.

Ipecacuanha (see ipecac earlier in this chapter) is a tincture one adds to water if the problems are nausea, vomiting and hypersalivation. *Carbo vegetabilis* is the one to grab if your stomach is bloated and you have gas. Phosphorous is for dizziness with a headache that has been made worse by warm weather. Tabacum is promoted for the type of motion sickness accompanied by a cold sweat that is relieved by cold, fresh air.

Again, I'd suggest that if you are thinking of trying any of these remedies, talk to your pregnancy care provider: Do not try to self-medicate. I find no data in the standard medical literature about the pros or cons of some of the remedies mentioned here.

Chapter 15

Purple Heart Motherhood

RUTH ANN

As I started writing this particular chapter, during a snow storm, I was contacted by a woman I had never met. Let's call her Ruth Ann. She had just learned that she was pregnant with her second child, almost 9 years after her first pregnancy, which had been complicated by hyperemesis gravidarum. She had been cared for at her local hospital, had required intravenous nutrition, and had been dreadfully sick until her emergency cesarean section at 34 weeks. Her daughter spend several weeks in the NICU (neonatal intensive care unit), but all turned out well in the end. Nonetheless, several of her care providers told her after the delivery that her case of hyperemesis gravidarum was the worst case they'd seen in years! Without advanced twenty-first century medical intervention, she would have died. There is no question in my mind about that.

Ruth Ann's desperate call to me was at 6 weeks, with a surprise pregnancy at age 45. A practicing, religious Catholic, she was also a nurse. We talked of all the aspects of her horrific prior morning-sickness/hyperemesis pregnancy—the tubes in her nose for feeding, the plastic tubes in her arm for intravenous nutrition, and how some of the factors in that pregnancy were not the same now. This pregnancy *could* be different, but there was certainly no guarantee. She wished desperately to be able to sleep through this pregnancy and wake up to have a wonderfully healthy child. Luck was temporarily on her side as she raced out to get Sea Bands and had 2 days of relief. A cold, snowy weekend rolled in with a barometric high, a change from the previous dreary, drizzly week. Walking in the crisp, clean, cold, fresh-smelling air brought relief—albeit temporary. When copious, metallic-tasting, thick saliva reappeared constantly, her course was down hill. She struggled to continue to be optimistic, but within a week she had made an appointment for an abortion. I was not totally surprised to get an e-mail message one morning when I logged on to my computer. She'd been through the ringer once already. Who would sign up to go through that again? I thought after our first chat. Having cared for many women who suffered from morning sickness every day for 9 months, I know at some point, some women will just call it quits. Men would never know how horrific it is unless someone had the unfortunate experience of being treated with chemotherapy or radiation therapy for cancer.

While triaging Ruth Ann by telephone and e-mail in the days leading up to her abortion decision, her struggle was apparent, and the enemy was clearly morning sickness. It was during these calls that by happenstance she got her nickname: Purple Heart Mom. She was doing battle with the morning-sickness war as countless thousands of women have over the centuries. Some women win the war of hyperemesis and can persevere until the natural course ends—anywhere from 12 to 40 weeks. You'll remember that the average gestational-age morning sickness goes away at 17.3 weeks, but 5 percent of morning-sick women are sick until delivery!

COMBAT DECORATION

Periodically, a woman loses some of her physical and mental health over chronic or intense morning sickness. Sad, but true, an untold number of women end up sacrificing the lives of their unborn children to end the misery. They can't understand why Mother Nature gives out horrible nausea and vomiting or why the medical establishment has not been able to find a solution to end this debilitating condition. By the time women are thinking, "this morning sickness has to end!" they feel there are few other options left to regain health and have a normal life and pregnancy. I've heard some women with morning sickness say they've seriously thought about suicide before abortion. Of course, they will rarely ever admit that to others. It is heart-wrenching to hear comments like these, but it's an indication to those in the care-providing world of just how miserable this situation is. It is so critical to continue the outreach for medical intervention and provide emotional support. One can never know when positive emotional support intersects with the natural end of morning sickness.

After years of caring for sick women, I have developed a few pretty strong opinions. I feel that women who suffer for the purpose of creating families deserve the Purple Heart of Motherhood. They endure something pretty awful: nausea and vomiting. The two villains (nausea and her side-kick vomiting) are what few other people ever endure for time ad infinitum, with the exception of course, cancer radiation and chemotherapy.

What is the Purple Heart? The Purple Heart was created by General George Washington on August 7, 1782, during the Revolutionary War. It is the oldest military decoration in the world in present use and was the first American award made available to the common soldier, initially created as the Badge of Military Merit. Our first president was greatly concerned about the well-being of his soldiers, and he often prayed with them. He had keen appreciation of the importance of the common soldier in any military campaign, especially those displaying outstanding valor and merit. Because there was no money to pay officers at this time, much less the average soldier, Washington created the Purple Heart for recognition. The original Purple Heart was designated to be awarded to members of the Armed Forces of the United States who were wounded by an instrument of war in the hands of the enemy. Posthumously, it is awarded to the next of kin in the name of any soldier killed in action or who died of wounds received in action. Although the original terms have been modified by the United States War Department, it is still today recognized specifically as a combat decoration. And, coincidentally, about the same time I finished the draft of this chapter, the United States Postal Service came out with Purple Heart stamps!

Although the wounds and injuries sustained in combat aren't really physically the same as those of morning-sickness women, I believe that morning-sickness women endure emotional or physical suffering (or both) that deserves similar understanding and recognition. Their struggle also warrants a call for more effective armor, in terms of research, medication, and treatment. When you finish reading this section on morning-sickness injuries, your understanding about what can happen with super-sized morning sickness might change. So, let's cruise through the medical archives.

WOUNDS OF MORNING SICKNESS
ABORTIONS

We might as well start at the beginning of the alphabet and the hardest situation for sick women to consider, and even harder for a lot of people to believe: abortion. The simple truth is that some women have abortions over morning sickness. This problem has had limited current investigation. The Motherisk Program in Toronto collected data from women who called with their desperate situations, looking for relief. They documented 17 of 1,100 callers (1.5 percent) in a 2-month period who just couldn't cope with out-of-control 24/7 hyperemesis any longer and chose abortions. They also noted 12 women who intended to terminate but didn't.

Motherisk investigators looked for differences between these two groups and a control group. All three groups were hospitalized, used antinausea/vomiting drugs, and had weight loss. The group who intended to abort but did not lost 18 pounds on average, was sick to 5.2 months, vomited an average of 7.3 times a day, and lost 64 days of work. The abortion group lost 13 pounds, lost an average of 20 work days, and chose abortion only to rid themselves of severe symptoms. Some women have said to me when they get admitted for care, "I've thought of suicide before abortion."

The Motherisk group in Toronto also studied the differences in attitude and management between hyperemesis women in Canada and the United States. They conducted a prospective, observational study and interviewed 1,444 women. Overall, they concluded that American women experience greater weight loss, had more hospitalizations, and lost more time at work than their Canadian counterparts. An astonishing 14 percent of Americans and 12 percent of Canadians reported that they had considered abortion because of their severe morning sickness, although the number who actually had abortions was much smaller.

Our hospital conducted a small study on morning sickness disability with the Boston Parents' Paper in 1998. Ours was a casual community survey in which women completed a form that allowed them to rate and rank two dozen suggested therapies on effectiveness for morning sickness, tell us know much money they lost, tell us whether they thought about abortion because of morning sickness, and tell us whether they limited their family size because of it. We also asked about sick-time loss. Of our 122 responses, two (1.6 percent) women acknowledged having an abortion. Eighteen women (14.7 percent) said they considered abortion, and 38 percent (46 women) said they limited family size because of morning sickness. Women wrote long letters, describing depression and anger about not having fun pregnancies and all wanting to know when we would find the cure.

Let's peruse the medical literature to see what situations might be candidates for the Purple Heart of Motherhood.

ACUTE KIDNEY FAILURE

In this 2002 case report, we have a 21-year-old woman who was admitted to an emergency room at 15 weeks into her second pregnancy. She was so dehydrated that her kidneys showed serious signs of damage and she required dialysis for 5 days to regain kidney function. She also had severe morning sickness in her first pregnancy and was hospitalized then as well. That pregnancy seemed to turn out okay; she delivered an 8 lb, 13 oz baby girl at term. What this woman weighed before her second pregnancy started was not reported. She was described as cachectic (malnourished or wasted in appearance) at 108 pounds. She hadn't urinated in days. For the first 5 days of this hospital admission, she was given aggressive intravenous fluids and only produced a small amount of urine. (I'd describe this woman as severely dehydrated—once a grape, now a raisin!)

In this case, an ultrasound showed a brain change in the developing baby. Whether or not this change was related to malnutrition in the mother is hard to know. At this point in time, this woman decided to have an abortion. The baby weighed 170 grams and had a large head but no other obvious defects. Eventually, the woman's kidney function returned, but only after 14 days of being hospitalized and treated aggressively with fluids.

DEATH

Hyperemesis gravidarum is a debilitating condition for pregnant women that, in rare cases, can result in death. Without proper medical attention, a pregnant woman can dehydrate or starve from chronic nausea and vomiting. Although a subject of debate in the medical community, some believe that Charlotte Bronte's death in 1855 was due to complications of severe morning sickness, specifically that she was dehydrated and could not eat (Weiss 1991). There is a case report of a woman in Japan who had a bleeding complication and eventually died (Wantanabe, Tanaka, and Masuda 1983). Her initial problem started out with morning sickness and progressed to a severe decrease in clotting factors, after which she bled to death.

ESOPHAGEAL RUPTURE

A ruptured esophagus is also called Boerhaave's Syndrome, after the doctor who first recognized this condition. The tube connecting the mouth to the stomach is called the esophagus. Most of the time food goes down this tube successfully and rarely does vomit comes back up the esophagus. Food is benign, but vomit is not. Vomit is highly acidic, semi–mashed-up food mixed with hydrochloric acid. If vomit is green, it's really bile. Bile is made by the liver and stored in the gallbladder, which is responsible for breaking down fat in the diet. Bile is made up of several components: bile acids, cholesterol, lecithin (lecithin is an agent that causes water to be able to mix with oil), bile pigments (coloring), and proteins.

For the stake of simplicity, remember bile is green and acidic. Some women vomit bile without eating anything. Retching is basically heaving or dry vomiting. Retching is a negative pressure situation. There is no food to return, but the vacuum produced by retching pulls out the next closest thing. That generally is bile sucked out of its storage chamber, the gallbladder. The thin esophagus, repeatedly exposed to acid, is weakened. Think of a weakened esophagus as a bald tire, and sooner or later—pop! You get a flat tire! Would it surprise you that some women have ruptured their esophagus? There are four reported cases since 1965. Who knows, there may be more that have not been written up and published in medical reports.

HEMORRHAGES

There are two case reports I found of bleeding disorders as a result of bad morning sickness. One report is from Japan and is not available in English, but according to the abstract, the woman died! The other case is a woman we cared for at the hospital where I work. She was identified with malnutrition the day she was admitted; she had had a significant weight loss and was dehydrated. The next day she had a profound nose bleed. This was the result of being deficient in vitamin K. With her nausea and vomiting, she was unable to eat foods high in vitamin K (e.g., green leafy vegetables), which are important for blood clotting.

Eyes

I've seen women who vomited so long and so hard that they have very bloodshot eyes. The force of vomiting can rupture fragile blood vessels in the eyes. In 1998, British doctors reported a situation in which a woman with severe morning sickness lost her vision. Prior to this catastrophe, she saw her doctors and was hospitalized briefly at 9 weeks into her third pregnancy with progressively worsening nausea and vomiting. She was also hospitalized at 11, 13, and 15 weeks. She was rehospitalized when she lost her sight at 17 weeks. An eye exam showed hemorrhages inside her retinas. At that time, an ultrasound revealed her baby had died in utero. She delivered the dead fetus.

Treated with thiamin and other vitamins and minerals, her vision partially returned. What is remarkable about this case is that it was only after she lost her sight that any indication of her nutritional status was identified. It is difficult to figure her prepregnancy weight, but there is an indication that she was obese. Nonetheless, she lost 12 kilograms, which is about 25 pounds.

This woman was also diagnosed with Wernicke's encephalopathy, which some considered just a thiamin deficiency. Nutritionally, dietitians would probably label this woman severely malnourished, having lost 14 to 16 percent of her original weight in 4 months, within a setting where weight gain is expected. Her vitamin and mineral status would be expected to be low but, that information was unavailable.

Eye sight is highly complex. Although most people will associate vitamin A with vision, vitamin A deficiency in young women is not likely unless there have been other long-term health problems before the pregnancy, such as gastrointestinal diseases, eating disorders, or excessive laxative use. Vitamin A is fat-soluble, and the body has long-term storage capability in fat tissue. The vision loss reported here was not due to a nutritional problem of vitamin A. This case is reported as a vision loss associated with the physical trauma of violent retching and vomiting. There is one case report of vision lost due to a diet deficient in vitamin B12, but, thankfully, there have been no reports of this problem occurring in pregnant women with bad morning sickness.

Also important for vision is that adequate calories or energy are consumed to help repair worn out tissues. The eye has many nerve endings, and the B-vitamins are important for nerve health. We can guess that this woman's nutritional status was not fabulous at the time. We know, however, that violent vomiting is a force known to disconnect nerve endings from the organs they are attached to. The next case will give you an indication of the violent force of vomiting.

SPLEEN

In 1995 there was a report in a Canadian surgical journal that a pregnant woman vomited so hard and for so long that she suffered a splenic avulsion. More simply put, her spleen had ripped away from its original location in her abdomen, and a hemorrhage resulted. She was into her third trimester when this event happened, and her fetus died.

PARALYSIS

A few years ago I reviewed a case of a woman who suffered permanent paralysis as a probable consequence of bad morning sickness. There are no reported cases in the literature similar to this, and I have only limited permission to report basic facts. To start, this woman was chronically dehydrated and lost weight because of her morning sickness and a few gaps in her care.

I learned a lot by reading this case, especially about the relationship between spinal fluid and urine output. In normal, healthy people, the rate of cerebrospinal fluid (the fluid that continues from the spinal cord to the brain) production is 0.3 to 0.4 milliliters per minute, which is about one-third the rate at which urine is produced, for a total about 2 cups a day.

If urine output is reduced, apparently spinal fluid production is also reduced. Some medical experts think that very thick spinal fluid can eventually become semisolid. The bottom line is that fluid in her spinal column got ultra-thick and formed an infarct, or a plug, in her spinal column. The nerves responsible for action signals to the legs were cut off at the pass, and signals could not be transmitted. The end result was paralysis from that point downward.

This rare disaster occurred at about 26 weeks, and the woman continued her pregnancy, resulting in her third healthy baby. As you might imagine, she had incredible health issues afterwards. And, tragically, the stress resulted in divorce. That's all I have permission to report; just know this is a true story (personal communication, Kidman, et al.). This woman is certainly a Purple Heart Mom.

SPONTANEOUS PNEUMOMEDIASTINUM

Pneumomediastinum is a condition in which air leaks from the lungs into the soft tissues around the heart and lungs. This air, in the wrong place, can compress the heart and lungs and cause pain as it collapses lung tissue. How it happens isn't really known. But there are two cases of this occurring in the setting of really bad morning sickness.

STARVATION

Let's review some fascinating brain facts, because it will help you to better appreciate how starvation and dehydration affect all living creatures.

The human brain is about 77 to 78 percent water, 10 to 12 percent fat, 8 percent protein, about 1 percent carbohydrate, about 1 percent inorganic salts, and 2 percent organic substances. The weight of the brain of an average 150-pound person is only 2 percent of a person's total weight, or 3 pounds. The brain needs glucose and oxygen to function—no ifs, ands, or buts about that! The brain uses 15 percent of the body's blood flow and uses 20 percent of the body's oxygen all the time. When a person is dehydrated and starving, the brain is doing the same thing, but very few people can see a brain losing weight because it is housed in the skull. That is both good and bad.

Weight loss can be a two-component situation: loss of real mass or loss of water. If one is well-hydrated, weight loss is predominantly body mass, whether fat or muscle. The brain is dependent upon calories to function. In a situation of low calorie intake, the body attempts to recycle a few calories to the brain by converting muscle to glucose (blood sugar) or from fat to make ketone bodies, a form of fat that the brain can use. A serious lack of energy to the brain results in mood or behavior changes as well as difficulty coordinating all the parts of the body. It is so important for the brain to get the energy it needs that in severe and prolonged starvation vital organ size is often reduced—that means the heart, the liver, the kidneys, and the pancreas.

Starvation simply is the prolonged lack of food, but it is often involuntary. Consider concentration-camp victims, dying to eat but having no access to food. Starvation in illness results in the same bodily sacrifice. Patients or victims of morning sickness want to eat, but something in their bodies prevents them from taking in adequate food, or food is found to be repulsive (nausea from morning sickness or chemotherapy) or is expelled from the body almost immediately (vomiting from morning sickness or diarrhea from gastrointestinal diseases).

Victims of anorexia nervosa can also be in a starvation mode, although they refuse to eat adequately for psychological reasons. Anorexia nervosa is complex; however, it should *not* be confused with hyperemesis gravidarum or the anorexia that often accompanies nausea and vomiting of pregnancy, or morning sickness. There are some women with anorexia nervous who get pregnant and have morning sickness on top of their past medical issues. Those situations can become complicated. However, 99.9 percent, or the majority of pregnant women, want to eat well and often because they know good nutrition is important for fetal development.

Let's talk about dieting for a minute. You or someone you know might have decided to try a crash diet in the hopes of getting into a great outfit for some special occasion. The dieter starts out enthusiastic, but gradually the dedication to the cause starts to dwindle. Consider any mood changes. Is the dieter cheerful? energetic? social? He or she probably is for 12 hours maximum or so. Everything is rosy until the hungry horrors set in. Ask a room of dieting people how pleasant the experience is. Not fun—in fact, painful and irritating—would be my guess as to how they would describe dieting. Consider that if dieting (starving) were so easy, we wouldn't have a country with staggering rates of obesity. Pure and simple, people avoid pain!

Few consider the fact that starving is painful when a pregnant woman complains of nausea and vomiting, has not eaten for days or weeks, and is losing weight. Please note again—starving is painful! Most people don't keep it up if they have a choice. Morning-sickness women often do not have a choice. Their nausea and vomiting prevents them from eating or keeping food down. Not eating means losing weight; losing weight means body changes and pain. This is simple biology 101. Starvation in pregnancy needs to be prevented, whatever its etiology or cause.

This section and the previous ones covered the non–brain damage complications of severe morning sickness. The next section, on Wernicke's encephalopathy and severe morning sickness (hyperemesis gravidarum), will show you what happens when nausea and vomiting become malignant and there is no or little early effective intervention.

WERNICKE'S ENCEPHALOPATHY

This review of literature on Wernicke's encephalopathy covers case reports from 1976 to fall 2002 only. There are countless more cases reports in the medical literature, going back as at least 1850, but I would expect those stories to parallel the ones detailed here.

Before delving into the case studies, I should provide some explanation of Wernicke's encephalopathy (WE). Carl Wernicke was the German who first identified the problem. *Encephalopathy* is a medical term that simply means a problem or disease of the brain. Wernicke's is most often considered as a disease associated with alcoholics, because it has been observed most often in the alcoholic population. Someone with WE may often be confused, have difficulty walking straight, and have a particular set of eye movements—going up and down or from side to side. This eye movement is called *nystagmus*.

Not all these symptoms have to occur together to have WE, but most in health care have been trained to expect these three symptoms together. WE initially was described as being caused by a lack of thiamin, which is vitamin B_1, but having a single nutrient deficiency all by itself rarely happens. Most modern clinical thinking suggests that WE is part of a complex situation of protein calorie malnutrition or encephalopathy of malnutrition. Cases of WE have been found in patients who have had stomach stapling for massive obesity; some cases have been documented in anorexia nervosa and in hyperemesis gravidarum. Consider the bottom line in all these situations: inadequate amounts of food to meet body (and brain) requirements. Wernicke's is pretty insidious; it comes on gradually, which is why sometimes cases get missed. Expect Wernicke's to evolve from poor nutrition and weight loss. Some people may be more predisposed to WE because of inherent genetic defects, but it's hard to identify who they are.

Although there have been many cases of WE in pregnant women, this section is based on 25 cases that I found in literature from 1976 to 2002. I will briefly discuss 5 of the 25 cases, which illustrate the global nature of the problem, and there will be a summary of all 25 cases at the end of the section. If you want to read more about the rest of the cases, check out the references at the end of this book and ask your librarian about interlibrary loans.

This situation happened in 1982 in Europe. A 20-year-old woman, pregnant for the first time, was hospitalized in her tenth week of pregnancy. She started her pregnancy at 181 pounds (82.5 kilograms), probably a bit overweight but we have no idea how tall she was. On admission to the hospital, they noted funny eye movements—rotary nystagmus. She continued to vomit up until her twentieth week of pregnancy, when she was transferred to another hospital. At week 20 she weighed 142 pounds (64.5 kilograms), a weight loss of 40 pounds in 20 weeks. She was described at this second hospital as "mildly confused, appeared overweight," and had problems with her short-term memory. She also had an in utero fetal demise (IUFD), or a dead baby. She delivered the baby; however, up to 4 months postpartum she had problems with her vision and her walking. (Nightingale, Bates, Heath, and Barron 1982)

A 22-year-old Irish woman in her second pregnancy was hospitalized in her seventeenth week of pregnancy with a history of 8 weeks of nausea and vomiting. We have no idea of her prepregnant weight, but, on admission to the hospital, she had lost almost 20 pounds (9 kilograms). She had a rapid pulse rate, which meant her heart was working really hard. She was disoriented, had difficulty walking, and had upward eye movements (vertical nystagmus). Fortunately, she was diagnosed with WE and treated with vitamins and fluids, which corrected her symptoms in 36 hours. (We have no idea whether she received nutrition.) She delivered a term baby boy weighing 7.4 pounds (3.4 kilograms). She did not have any vision, memory, or walking problems thereafter. (Flannelly, Turner, Connolly, and Stronge 1990)

Just so you don't think WE is just a European problem, let's go to Japan. In 1994 an 18-year-old woman 8 weeks into her first pregnancy was hospitalized. She'd been sick for 6 weeks. We have no idea how much she weighed before she got pregnant, but at 8 weeks she was 101 pounds (46 kilograms). Nineteen weeks later she was transferred to another hospital, weighing 84 pounds (38 kilograms). Her albumin (a blood protein) level was 2.8 milligrams per deciliter.

She had difficulty walking and standing. The hospital drew her blood to determine her thiamin status. Her thiamin was low, and other markers suggested that metabolic acidosis was occuring. A CAT scan of her brain showed brain changes consistent with starvation. At week 21, her baby was found to have died in her uterus. For at least 2 months, she needed to walk with two canes and had memory problems. (Ohkoshi, Ishii, and Shoji 1994)

From Scandinavia there was a report from 1999 in which a 25-year-old woman was seen at 11 weeks into her third pregnancy. She had had no live children yet. No information was given about how long she'd been sick. She was found to be anemic and had elevations in specific liver function tests. She also had (EEG) electro encephalogram changes. The hospital staff reported that she was apathetic, had confabulation (means making up stories), couldn't walk straight, was disoriented, had "ocular disturbances," was inattentive, had no short-term memory, and had no ankle or knee reflexes. An MRI (magnetic resonance image) showed brain changes. She was diagnosed with WE and treated with vitamins; her symptoms started to disappear within 48 hours. At 40 weeks, she delivered a baby boy, who apparently was healthy. Postpartum, the woman had vision problems. (Gardian, Voros, Jardanhazy, Ungurean, and Vecsei 1999)

In 2001 doctors in Turkey reported a case of a 25-year-old woman in her second pregnancy with WE. She had nausea and vomiting in her first pregnancy, but more details were not available for that pregnancy. In the second pregnancy, she was seen at 10 weeks and had been sick for an estimated 6 weeks. She had a preexisting overactive thyroid condition for which she was taking medication. On admission, she had elevated liver functions. She was also described as being confused, having no short-term memory, being apathetic, behaving as though she was very sleepy, exhibiting up-down and side-to-side eye movements, and having no deep tendon reflexes in her legs. An MRI was done, and brain changes were found. She was promptly treated with vitamins. Her treatment continued until she delivered a healthy baby at term. Postpartum, she had no problems. (Togay-Isikay, Yigit, and Mutluer 2001)

There are compartments in the brain known as ventricles, which are like holes filled with fluid. A person with WE tends to have more fluid in these holes. The question to be asked is why is there more fluid? Maybe the brain matter around the ventricles shrinks such that proportions of solid tissue and fluid change. A starved brain loses weight. Consider this analogy: Does the hole in a doughnut get bigger, or does the doughnut get smaller? Think about maintaining body tissues; you need calories and all sorts of nutrients. Brain changes could simply be starvation changes. And in order to regain brain function, one needs to prevent a low-calorie situation and refeed all the important nutrients to build tissues. These include all the vitamins and minerals, as well as the right fats and protein.

Of the 25 cases I researched on WE as a complication of severe morning sickness, the outcomes of pregnancy were not good. Forty percent of the cases had spontaneous abortions, miscarriages, or IUFD. Twelve percent of the women decided to have abortions. Seventy-six percent of these women continued to have some problems after the pregnancy was over—memory loss, vision problems, or difficulty walking.

Now you have the answers to that question "so how bad can morning sickness get?" Pretty bad, don't you agree? I'm sure there are countless others out there who also deserve the Purple Heart of Motherhood!

Chapter 16

Medications

NELL

Years ago I worked with an African American woman who was pregnant with her fourth child. Working in food services is really hard when you have morning sickness. Nell didn't complain much about being queasy, but she would excuse herself frequently from the floor kitchen before and after sending out trays to patients. I figured it was the hot galley getting to her.

One day I looked at Nell and thought she was going to faint—she had broken out into a sweat. That's when she told me she was pregnant and sick. This was not new for her—just pretty stale! She felt this pregnancy was worse than the others, and she wasn't sure whether it was related to her type of work or not.

I lent her a copy of my morning sickness book, and she suggested that more information on drugs would be helpful in future books. Nell also asked what herbs might be helpful. Her mother was living with her family for a short while to help out and was interested in herbal medicine.

About that same time, I was heading out of town to a big nutrition conference in Denver. My traveling friend and colleague, Ms. Patsy, and I had plans to drive to Santa Fe and Taos after the conference so I could try to interview Native Americans about what sort of remedies they might use for morning sickness. That was a great plan, but, in fact, finding women with Native American backgrounds and stories from their grandmothers was not so easy. Instead, I bought all the books I could find on herbs along the way.

There were lists of herbs to try for various stages of pregnancy. The one that seemed to pop up the most was catnip tea. Once I was back, Nell asked me what I'd unearthed from my interviews. I told her I'd come up empty-handed, but a few books had suggested catnip tea. I was still up to my ears in books, so I told her I would let her know what else I found.

A few days later, Nell announced, "I'm cured!" She said she'd gone home and told her mother what I'd read, and her mother promptly went out and found a particular brand of catnip tea. Every night for 4 nights, her mom would make her a cup of catnip tea before she went to sleep. Every night for 4 nights, Nell held it down successfully and slept like a baby once again. "Okay," I thought, maybe the catnip tea worked; after all, it is a relative of mint, according to my books. Or maybe Nell hit that magic day when she was going to be over morning sickness. It is hard to know for sure, but she was grateful nonetheless.

That episode was a while ago, and I hardly gave it a second thought until the third week in September 2003. I gave myself a day off from writing and drove to Plum Island, north of Boston, with a picnic lunch and a book, *The Nine Emotional Lives of Cats*. Now, you might be asking, what do that book and Nell have in common? The answer is catnip. What I learned was that *Nepeta cataria*, the official name of catnip is related to marijuana and contains the chemical nepetalactone in its stems and leaves! What exactly was in Nell's tea? Given that botanical agents were really the basis of medicines years ago, we've now evolved to twenty-first century medications. Research on nausea reduction and vomiting prevention has looked for active ingredients in both plants and manufactured medicine that might alter activity in the vomiting center of the brain. For example, Marinol, a relative of the active ingredient in marijuana, has been used to relieve nausea.

As you might recall from previous chapters, researchers have found higher levels of some of the pregnancy hormones in women who have more severe morning sickness. So too much of a natural thing is not necessarily healthy. And because hormones are produced internally, you can't take them out of the body to reduce their concentration. This essentially leaves one medical option for pregnant women: We can use medications to try to mitigate the consequences of the elevated hormones (e.g., nausea and vomiting).

MEDICATIONS FOR MORNING SICKNESS

You know, of course, that your doctor is the only person who should be prescribing medications to you, pregnant or not. Never, ever self-medicate. Any herbals concoctions should be reviewed with your doctor as well. Adverse reactions have been reported between botanical and pharmaceuticals.

The Food and Drug Administration (FDA) classifies drugs according to an alphabetic system of risks: A, B, C, and D. The higher the letter, the fewer studies have been done, so more caution is exercised. For obvious ethical reasons, there is no direct research done on pregnant women.

You should always check out any medication you might be taking for the latest updates. This book obviously cannot provide updates on events that might occur. The purpose of this chapter is not to prescribe medication but simply to give you information to discuss with your doctor. Credible sources of Internet drug information can be accessed through www.entrezpubmed.org. You can also check out the National Library of Medicine, Micromedex Inc., and WebMD.

SEROTONIN ANTAGONISTS

These drugs are considered 5-HT3 receptor antagonists and work on the vagus nerve, the CTZ (chemoreceptor trigger zone), and the gut. They are category B drugs.

There are three drugs in this group: Zofran (Ondanestron), Kytril (Granisetron), and Anzemet (Dolasetron). Only Zophran has been used in hyperemesis. It's an expensive drug. It is available as an oral form, an intravenous form, and a suppository. Dosing ranges from 4 to 8 milligrams every 6 hours.

CORICOSTEROIDS

There are concerns about how much and when to use corticosteroids because they cross the placenta. The following drugs need to be tapered over several weeks if they are used:

Methylprednisolone, a pregnancy category C drug
Prednisone, a category B drug
Cortisone, category D drug.

The range for Methylprednisolone is 48 milligrams per day for 3 to 5 days, followed by a slow tapering over 2 to 3 weeks. Steroids are tough on maternal bones, so an adequate calcium diet is important.

ANTIHISTAMINES

Antihistamines are category B drugs. Included here are Bonine, Antivert, Marezine, Dramamine (Dimenhydrinate), and Doxylamine (Unisom). Also in this category are Benadryl, Tigan, Vistaril, and Atarax.

Unisom was part of the medication Bendectin used in the 1970s and 1980s as an anti–morning sickness drug. Also part of Bendectin was vitamin B_6. Bendectin has been resurrected in Canada and travels under the name Declectin. Dosing for common antihistamines are as follows:

Declectin: 1 tablet in the morning, 1 at mid-day, and 2 at night
Unisom: 1/2 to 1 tablet at night (ask your doctor before taking additional dosages)
Dramamine (used for motion sickness): ranges from 50 to 100 milligrams every 4 to 6 hours

The side effects of the antihistamines are drowiness, blurred vision, dry mouth, constipation, urinary retention, restlessness, upset stomach, nervousness, and headache. You might not feel a heap better after taking these, but if you sleep, you'll be able to forget how miserable you are! Sleep provides relief!

ANTIDOPAMINERGICS (PHENOTHIAZINES)

Anitidopaminergics, or phenothiazines, are category C drugs. An antidopaminergic blocks the action of dopamine, a neurotransmitter in the brain that is thought to relax muscles in the gastrointestinal tract. These agents have side effects of drowiness, dry mouth, low blood pressure, constipation, urinary retention, extrapyramidal symptoms (means you have a tough time walking and might be really shaky), restlessness, confusion, and fatigue. (Doesn't that make you feel great?)

Agents here include Compazine, Stemetil, Phenergen, Thorazine, and Haldol. All these agents are available in oral, intravenous, and intramuscular forms. Compazine and Thorazine are also available as suppositories.

Zantac (Ranitidine), Pepcid (Famotidine), and Prevacid (Lansoprazole) are also used. Tagamet (Cimetidine), however, is not recommended in pregnancy because of antiandrogenic effects (meaning they can cause reproductive anomalies or altered sex organ characteristics) that have been observed in research on animals.

PROKINETIC AGENTS

Prokinetics are category B drugs. They work by blocking certain receptors in the CTZ (chemoreceptor trigger zone), increasing the CTZ threshold, and decreasing the sensitivity of the visceral (internal) nerves that send signals from the gut to the vomiting center in the brain. Included in this category are Reglan, Maxeran, and Propulside (Cisapride).

Side effects include drowsiness, dizziness, abdominal pain, diarrhea, restlessness, depression, and a shaky feeling. You might want to check out any medication with OTIS. OTIS is the Organization of Teratology Information Services, which has a database of all medications and environmental agents as well as lists of any birth defects and safety concerns. Find them on the Internet at www.otispregnancy.org. They also have national toll-free numbers: (866) 626-OTIS (or 6847). This is a fabulous, free service. In Massachusetts, their number is (781) 487-2386.

OTHER MEDICATIONS TO CONSIDER

For Emetrol (a fructose, dextrose, and phosphoric acid solution), take 1 to 2 tablespoons every 3 hours. I was unable to find any literature on how this medication actually works. A few years ago I called the company who now owns this product, and they had no information to give me. I guess if coke syrup works, this might work in the same way.

Marinol (Dronabinol) is a marijuana derivative. The dose has not been established in severe morning sickness. A few years ago we had two women with severe hyperemesis on the unit. One was thin and pregnant with twins; the other one was obese. Both had lost several pounds. Each woman had a different doctor, and both were prescribed Marinol after everything else failed. The Marinol worked for Mrs. Twins but not for the other woman. The reason for this has not been determined. Perhaps we should have tried giving them catnip tea.

Powdered ginger supplements can be taken at 250 milligrams four times a day. Be aware that the efficacy of these products may vary depending on how long they've been sitting around. One study from Thailand using handmade ginger supplements suggested that they work in mild cases. However, I learned from the chief investigator that they did not include severe cases in their study.

MEDICATIONS TO AVOID

Anticholinergics and antispasmodics should not be used during pregnancy. This includes scopolmine and belladonna.

Valium is considered a category D drug, and no dose has been established for pregnancy.

Droperidol (Inapsine) has been used in hyperemesis but was taken off the market because of serious problems in the elderly and critically ill, intensive-care patients.

MEDICINAL REMINDERS

In my clinical experience, having an adequate fluid intake, whether by mouth or by vein seems to help a lot when medications are used, in addition to correcting those electrolytes mentioned in Chapter 11.

Don't forget to take prenatal vitamins and calcium! Again, be sure to keep all medications out of the reach of children and pets.

Appendix

In this appendix, you will find information about relevant Web sites of organizations and groups that offer support to women suffering from morning sickness, a discussion of some specific conditions or allergies that may contribute to sickness, and names of special foods and health products, as well as their suppliers, that may help mitigate symptoms of morning sickness. Not everyone has access to computers and the Internet, so I've added phone and fax numbers with addresses when they are available.

USEFUL CHARTS

To help you keep tabs on your weight during morning sickness, you can record your weight on the Weight Change Chart (Figure A.1) and plot that information on the grid provided in Figure A.2 for each week of your pregnancy.

The fluid chart in Figure A.3 will help you keep a record of your daily fluid intake. You can write in the type of fluid (water, tea, juice, etc.) above the cup and indicate the amount that you drank. Make several

Figure A.1

WEIGHT CHANGE CHART

date of last menstrual cycle:_____
prepregnancy weight:_____ date:_____
due date:_____ (dated by your M.D.)
Begin dating this chart by the dates your doctor gives you. This may be two weeks
different from your particular dates. Doctors have been dating from a lunar calendar
for centuries, and this is not about to change soon! You can make another copy of this
chart if you wish, to use according to *your* method before your first prenatal visit.

Week No.	Date	New Weight	Change from Last Week	Comments
1				
2				
3				
4				
5				
6				
7				
8				
9				
10				
11				
12				
13				
14				
15				
16				
17				
18				
19				
20				
21				
22				
23				
24				
25				
26				
27				
28				
29				
30				
31				
32				
33				
34				
35				
36				
37				
38				
39				
40				
41				
42	(overdue!)			

Figure A.2

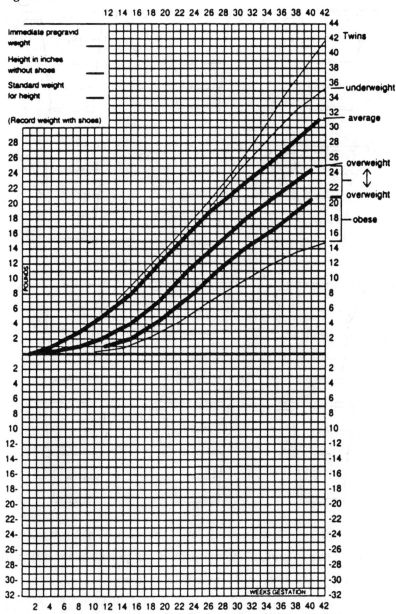

Pattern of normal prenatal gain in weight.
Source: Adapted from U.S. Department of health Education and Welfare, Social and Rehabilitation Service, Children's Bureau.

Figure A.3

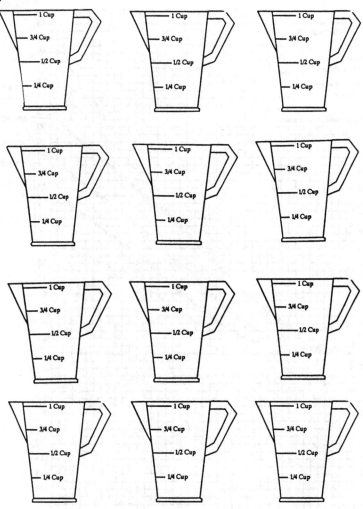

copies of this page, one for every day of the week. When you see your doctor, be sure to bring along this data. It will provide ammunition to help justify the need for intravenous fluids at home.

MEDICAL RESOURCES

1. www.healthfinder.gov (United States Department of Health and Human Services) The healthfinder Web site will help you

locate virtually *anything* you want to know about medicine and health.

2. www.fns.usda.gov/fncs/(Food Nutrition Services of the United States Department of Agriculture) Start here to learn about the WIC (Women, Infants, and Children) supplemental nutrition program and determine whether you are eligible.

3. www.hon.ch (Health On the Net Foundation) The Health On the Net Foundation in Geneva, Switzerland, strives to improve international health by providing information to the general public and the medical community on the Internet.

4. www.ncahf.org (National Council Against Health Fraud, Inc.) Before you fall victim to any health products or services that sound too good to be true, log onto this site and do some investigation. Medical scams are as plentiful as ants at a picnic! You can sign up online to receive the Consumer Health Digest, or you can write to the National Council Against Health Fraud at 119 Foster Street, Building R, Second Floor, Peabody, MA 01950. This newsletter is written by antifraud guru Stephen Barrett, MD, who has been protecting consumers for years.

5. www.nih.gov (National Institutes of Health) The NIH Web site provides links to late-breaking medical news and a variety of other health information. You can also access unedited text of consumer health publications.

6. www.ncbi.nlm.nih.gov/pubmed/ (National Library of Medicine) If you've read about a study and want more details, this is the place to start digging. Be aware that this site does provides citations and abstracts (when available) to journal articles, but it does not provide the full article text. In many cases, a fee will be required to retrieve the complete article.

7. www.navigator.tufts.edu (Tufts University Nutrition) The navigator provides something for everyone—professionals,

consumers, and educators. This is a wonderful Web site, chock-full of practical advise and easy-to-understand results of new studies.

8. http://www.dietitian.com (Ask the Dietitian) My friend Joanne Larsen created this site years ago; it provides a host of great information.

9. www.marchofdimes.com (The March of Dimes) The March of Dimes (MOD) site provides all sorts of information about preventing birth defects and premature deliveries. There are MOD offices in most all states to provide local help.

10. www.visembryo.com (The Visible Embryo) This is a Web site where you can follow fetal development. Some specialized Web sites can provide you with more information on pregnancy complications.

11. www.about.com The About.com Web sites give information on virtually any topic you might want to know about, including gestational diabetes and stress.

12. www.sidelines.org (Sidelines National Support Network) This is your lifeline if you are bedridden or have a high-risk pregnancy. Sidelines matches you with a volunteer who has had a complicated pregnancy and will give you emotional support by calling you on the phone or sending you e-mail on a regular basis. Sidelines also has a bookstore for pregnancy materials. If you want more information but don't have Internet access, you can call (888) 477-4754.

13. www.motherisk.org (Motherisk) This is a premier site for morning sickness help. Motherisk is a Canadian organization at the Hospital for Sick Children in Toronto. It is funded by the Duchesnay pharmaceutical company from Laval (in Quebec) Canada. Motherisk does morning-sickness counseling over the

phone in English and French. You can reach them by phone at (800) 436-8477.

14. www.lamaze.org (Lamaze International) Lamaze International promotes education about lamaze and normal childbirth. If you don't have Internet access, you can call (800) 368-4404 for more information.

For help and information in the months to come, check out the following sites:

Healthy kids	www.keepkidshealthy.com (Keep Kids Healthy)
	www.kidshealth.org (KidsHealth, part of the Nemours Foundation)
	www.zerotothree.org (Zero to Three: National Center for Infants, Toddlers, and Families)
Adoption	www.adoption.about.com (About.com)
Pregnancy loss	www.hygeia.org (Hygeia Foundation) phone: (203) 387-3589 fax: (203) 387-3589
Down syndrome	www.ndss.org (National Down Syndrome Society) phone: (800) 221-4602 fax: (212) 979-2873
Alcohol and substance abuse	www.motherisk.org (Motherisk)
Genetics	www.nsgc.org (National Society of Genetic Counselors)
Breastfeeding	www.lalecheleague.org (La Leche League International) phone: (800) LALECHE (523-3243)
Infant nutrition	www.fns.usda.gov/wic (Women, Infants, and Children Program) phone: (703) 305-2746
Single parents	www.singlerose.com (Single Rose)
	www.singleparentcentral.com (Single Parent Central)

Multiple births	www.mostonline.org (Mothers of Supertwins) phone: (631) 859-1110 www.tripletconnection.org (Triplet Connection) phone: (209) 474-0885 fax: (209) 474-9243
Thyroid disease	www.thyroid.about.com (About.com)
Depression	www.depressionafterdelivery.com (Depression After Delivery) phone: (800) 944-4773
Vaginal birth after cesarean	www.vbac.com (VBAC.com)

EMOTIONAL RESOURCES

There are a few Web sites available for women with severe cases of morning sickness.

1. www.members.cox.net/tcarpenter3/main (Hyperemesis Gravidarum Awareness Page)
2. www.hyperemesis.org (HER Foundation)
3. www.morningsickness.net (my morning sickness Web site)

Chat rooms can also be helpful for emotional support. Support chat rooms exist for virtually every need. There are chat rooms for women who have terminated pregnancies because they could not find relief from their horrible hypermesis. There are also chat rooms for hypermesis gravidarum survivors. Delphi Forums is one of the many sites where you can find support chat rooms. Although it is good that support like this exists, it is unfortunate that we haven't yet found a way to provide relief for all the women who suffer.

You can also order CDs on stress management. And don't forget to check out your local library's audio collection.

SPIRITUAL GUIDANCE

Although *The Anatomy of Hope: How People Prevail in the Face of Illness* is not about morning sickness, it is about finding a real hope that one will survive the current ordeal. I was fortunate enough to hear Dr. Jerome Groopman read from his fabulous work in the dreadful cold winter of 2004. He spoke eloquently about "exiting a labyrinth of pain" and the "biology of hope." Researchers are now discovering that there are biochemical changes that take place in the body when one is hopeful—and those changes can make a world of difference. If you don't have the energy to read the whole book, at least read the section called "The Body-Mind and Mind-Body Connection: The Risk of a Vicious Cycle."

In Larry Dossey's masterpiece book, *Healing Words: The Power of Prayer and the Practice of Medicine,* he starts every chapter off with quotes to live by. Starting the chapter, "How to Pray and What to Pray For" is this poignant quotation from the late Duke Ellington: "Everyone prays in their own language, and there is no language that God does not understand."

H. PYLORI

This nasty stomach bug has been found in some women with morning sickness. It's more common in underdeveloped countries where food sanitation is lacking; however, a few of my patients have tested positive for it in Boston. Left untreated, it can go on to produce a wickedly bad case of ulcers. Treatment is often with antibiotics, which can be a scenario similar to dog chasing its tail if taking pills makes you throw up!

New research suggests that having a diet that contains fermented dairy products—containing the culture known as *Lactobacillus johnsonii*—might reduce the incidence of H. *pylori* in the first place. A chronic H. *pylori* infection is a risk factor for gastric cancer, which is why it needs to be treated. Other researchers have looked at the relationship with a diet high in antioxidant nutrients from fruits and vegetables that appear to protect the stomach.

FOOD SENSITIVITIES

In recent years, interest in a relatively new allergy to latex rubber has soared. Adverse reactions range from mild skin redness to touching a product with latex to severe respiratory complaints and on rare occasion, death. Researchers have recently found a connection between certain tropical fruits and latex, the white sticky fluid that comes from the rubber-tree plant. They may have closely related proteins or peptides. For this reason, the syndrome has been given the name of latex-diet syndrome or latex-fruit syndrome. Not everyone with a latex sensitivity will have a problem with food, but we want to acquaint you with some of the foods the might be considered close relatives to the latex plant.

An individual's response to foods may vary widely, so please keep that in mind. Some signs of intolerance include headache, itchy mouth, tight throat, difficulty breathing, stomachache, blotchy skin, or red patches. This list provides you with names of some foods that are suspects in the latex-diet syndrome.

High probability: Banana, avocado, and chestnut
Moderate probability: Apple, carrot, celery, tomato, papaya, kiwi,
    potato, melon, and mango

Low or undetermined probability: Pear, peach, cherry, pineapple, strawberry, mugwort, soybean, fig, grape, walnut, apricot, passion fruit, peanut, spinach, and beets (Pregnant women should avoid mugwort, or Artemisia vulgaris, regardless of whether or not they have latex allergies because it can cause uterine contractions.)

Digestive enzymes available as over-the-counter aids may also contain compounds from pineapple and papaya. Bromelin is found in pineapple, whereas papain is found in papaya. Besides being used as digestive enzymes, these compounds can also be found in meat tenderizers. These may pose a problem for highly sensitive latex-diet persons.

Also keep in mind that when fruits are harvested, workers may be wearing latex-coated gloves. A food you react to may not contain naturally related latex peptides or proteins but may have picked up latex particles somewhere along the way to your dinner table.

Latex gloves are commonly used by employees in preparing foods so, for those who are particularly allergic to latex, eating out might present problems unless you discuss your allergy with restaurant personnel. Most hospitals, of course, do not allow the use of latex gloves in food services.

Some persons with asthma and other respiratory problems find that eating raw fruits and vegetables causes difficulty, whereas eating cooked or peeled fruit does not. Pollen, which sticks to the skins of fruits, may be part of the problem. Cooking inactivates most pollen. This may explain why a cooked food may be better tolerated compared to its raw counterpart.

My suggestion to anyone who has a food allergy is this: Wear a medic-alert bracelet that lists your food allergies, name, phone number, doctor, and emergency phone numbers. When an emergency happens, time is of the essence. And, as always, tell your health care team about *all* your allergies.

SPECIAL PRODUCT RESOURCES

LACTOSE-REDUCED BEVERAGES

Kefir with FOS (fructooligosaccharides) is a fermented dairy product that has active cultures for the health of your gastrointestinal tract. Kefir has milk proteins in it. It is considered a probiotic, which means that the active ingredients help restore the good bacteria that is important for digestion of some foods. Some women react to various medications with new onset diarrhea; these beverages might be helpful in this instance. Kefir comes in various flavors. I found two brands at Whole Foods Market: Helios and Lifeway. No Web site is available fom Lifeway at the time of this writing, but the Web site for Helios is www.heliosnutrition.com.

You're probably wondering what in the world an FOS is. FOS's are considered functional foods, which are foods with enhanced nutritional properties. FOS is an indigestible carbohydrate that occurs naturally in many fruits, vegetables, and grains in small amounts. Food producers concentrate FOS into various foods to enhance health benefits. FOS has been associated with reducing pathological bacteria in the large colon, reducing free radical formation, restoring healthy gut bacteria, and increasing the production of B-complex vitamins.

NONDAIRY BEVERAGES

Rice milk is a great partner with your breakfast cereal. Be aware that rice milk is not generally a great source of protein. It has only 1 gram of protein per 8-ounce serving, but can provide 25 percent of the recommended daily intake (RDI) of calcium and vitamin D if it is fortified. Compare this to cow's milk with 8 grams of protein per 8-ounce serving.

Soy milk is another beverage for the person looking for a cow's milk alternative. It has 7 grams of protein per 8 ounces and contains various fortified nutrients. Pay attention to whether you are purchasing soy milk or *soy milk drink*. Soy milk *drink* has about half the protein of soy milk, only 4 grams per 8 ounces. Both will work to moisten your breakfast cereal or as a base to make a fruit smoothie.

Soya powder is available so you can make your own soy milk as needed. One quarter cup of dry mix will provide 10 grams of soy protein. It can be purchased from Fearn Natural Foods in Mequon, Wisconsin. Fearn Natural Foods also produces soya granules; a half-cup serving has an impressive 22 grams of protein. Recipes are provided on the packaging.

Oat milk (yes, oat—not goat!) from Pacific Foods is another option. You can find their Web site at www.pacificfoods.com. Pacific Foods also offers a multigrain nondairy beverage with 5 grams of protein per 8-ounce serving.

Goat milk is available as an instant powder from Meyenberg ([800] 343-1185 or www.meyenberg.com). The Meyerberg product has folic acid added. Not all goat milk has folic acid, so you need to be sure to ask especially. The lack of folic acid makes unfortified goat milk an unsuitable product to feed babies and growing children.

Snapple-a-Day is a meal replacement product. This beverage is Kosher, lactose free, and has 7 grams of soy protein per 11.5-ounce serving, with 100 percent of your RDI for vitamins A, C, E and 25 percent of many other vitamins and calcium. It does not have to be refrigerated until you open it, which is part of its appeal. You can store this in your desk and pour it over ice to sip when you need it. An 11.5-ounce serving provides 210 calories. This is one-eighth of most women's daily needs.

OTHER BEVERAGES

Organic Fruit Squeezies from Walnut Acres are fruit juices in tubes that you freeze and eat in frozen form. For more info go to www.strength.org or call 1-800-969-4767.

By the way, this company donates part of their profits to antihunger organizations like Share Our Strength (SOS).

Optimize is a high-calcium, clear, liquid beverage. The flavor I tried was strawberry-kiwi, which was a bit sweet, but adding a slice of lemon or lime could mitigate the sweetness. A 10-ounce serving provides 50 percent (500 mg) of the RDI for calcium, 44 percent for vitamin K, and 100 percent for vitamin D. It also contains some magnesium and vitamin C. There is no protein in this product. It is made by Nature Made Nutritional Products of Mission Hills, California. For more information go to www.optimizenutrition.com or call (800) 669-9163.

ReVital Squeezers is a pediatric electrolyte solution. The delivery system is a plastic bottle with a built-in straw. All you have to do is snip the straw and sip. This seems to be a good solution when you need some fluids on the go or in the office. You could keep 1 or 2 of these in the refrigerator in the office for emergencies at work.

GLUTEN-FREE AND WHEAT-FREE PRODUCTS

Fearn Natural Foods in Mequon, Wisconsin, offers a rice baking mix and a brown-rice baking mix. Fearn Natural Foods is only one source of soya powder. I happened on this product and was pleased to find that they included recipes on use. Sometimes people who are new to vegetarianism are timid about how to use alternative protein foods and need some recipe and menu directions at the time of purchase.

Lotus Foods offers a Bhutanese red rice flour. Find them at www.worldofrice.com or fax them at (510) 525-4226.

Pamela's Products sells gluten-free ginger cookies with sliced almonds. Call (707) 462-6605 to find the nearest outlets to you or find them online at www.pamelasproducts.com.

EssenSmart makes a sweet ginger soy cookie for vegans, a gluten-free lemon poppyseed cookie, and a cinnamon cookie that is egg-free.

Ancient Harvest produces Quinoa (pronounced keen-wa). This grain is a gluten-free product that has 5 grams of protein per half-cup serving and 10 percent RDI for iron.

Edward and Sons' puts out a brown-rice snap (cracker) that contains no wheat.

GINGER

NewChapter's Maple-Ginger Tonic is Vermont maple syrup blended with their own supercritical ginger extract. It contains 20 percent of pungent ginger compounds and 4 percent ziniberene. You can take 1 to 2 teaspoons straight from the container and mix it into sparking water or hot water for your own ginger ale or ginger tea, respectively. Find out more from New Chapter by writing to 22 High Street, Brattleboro, VT 05301, calling (800) 543-7279, or visiting their Web site at www.newchapter.info.

HEALTH AND BEAUTY AIDS

Women often complain about health and beauty aids and how powerful the fragrances have become. It really isn't the fragrance that has increased in potency, it is that phenomena of the "radar nose"—courtesy of rising estrogen levels—that drives women with morning sickness crazy.

The items listed here are certainly not the only products in the aroma-reduced department, but I've sample many of them and I think they are worth your consideration:

Tom's of Maine (www.tomsofmaine.com) makes toothpaste, soaps, and other cosmetics.

Natural homeopathic-style baking soda toothpaste is unflavored and contains calcium.

Natural ginger-mint toothpaste is my favorite. It comes in fluoride and fluoride-free versions.

Natural fennel-flavored toothpaste is good if you like licorice.

Natural glycerin bar soap (unscented) and liquid natural glycerin soap are two alternatives to regular bar and liquid soaps.

GROCERY STORES

If you don't live close to a Whole Foods Market (WFM), you can access their offerings online and probably save yourself a lot of running round and expense, especially if you live in a rural area. WFM is essentially a health-food grocery store, but it also sells lots of new products, books, and even cosmetics. The items are more expensive than standard grocery stores, but the focus is on very healthy, fresh foods. They have one of the biggest supplies of food for people with allergies. Gluten-free, lactose-free, and peanut-free diets can all be serviced by this chain. Their stores can ship hard-to-get products to clients with special needs. Reach them online at www.wholefoodsmarket.com.

Trader Joe's is another chain with a Web site that has specialty products, including gluten-free, kosher, and dairy-free offerings. Check them out online at www.traderjoes.com or call (800) SHOP-TJS.

ORGANIC FOOD

Information from the Environmental Working Group, a nonprofit group based in Washington, D.C., recommends that we eat organic fruits and vegetables, especially off-season. If you cannot buy organic, consider buying locally. Most produce grown overseas will contain higher levels of pesticides and ripening agents than similar ones grown locally, even if the local products are not organic. In recent studies, the highest amounts of pesticides were found on conventionally grown apples, apricots, bell peppers, cantaloupe, celery, cherries, green beans, peaches, spinach, and strawberries. Buying organic reduces your level of pesticide exposure. When buying nonorganic fruits and vegetables, thoroughly scrub them under running water to remove traces of pesticides from their skins and crevices.

Here are a few definitions for organic foods that will help you shop for more healthful foods:

The term *100 percent organic* means that the product must contain only organically produced raw or processed material, excluding water and salt. The name of the certifying agent *must* appear on packages, and the use of its certifying seal is optional. The use of the United States Department of Agriculture (USDA) organic seal is also optional.

Organic means that the product must contain at least 95 percent organically produced ingredients. The label must state the percentage of organic ingredients and the name of the certifying agent. The use of the USDA organic seal is optional.

Made with organic ingredients means that at least 70 percent of the product's ingredients must be organic.

RELIABLE NUTRITION PUBLICATIONS

The Web sites www.askthedietitian.com and www.dietitian.com will take you to great Web resources and allow you to ask all sorts of health and nutrition questions.

For pennies a week, you can subscribe to health newsletters and get quality nutrition and health information without any advertisements. Newsletters are portable and great to read while commuting. They are also easy to share with friends and neighbors. Quality health newsletters generally include something for all age groups in each issue.

Nutrition Alert publishes six issues a year at a cost of $15. The editor is Elizabeth Somers, MA, RD (author of several quality nutrition books). I love this newsletter. My favorite section is the one that discusses the latest global studies about nutrition and diet issues. Write to 4742 Liberty Road South, PMB 148, Salem, Oregon 97302 to subscribe.

Elizabeth Somer has also written a fabulous book on nutrition during pregnancy, which I highly recommend. It is called *Nutrition for a Healthy Pregnancy*, 2nd edition. This book has a lot of practical advice and easy-to-fix recipes to make eating healthy a no-brainer.

Prevention Magazine publishes 12 issues a year at a cost of $15. This magazine is a great size (5 by 8 inches) if you are commuting. They also have a Web page with links, and they will personally answer your questions. Find them at www.prevention.com or write to this address: c/o Rodale publication at 33 E. Minor Street, Emmaus, PA 18098.

Environmental Nutrition has been providing useful nutrition advice for over 30 years. They publish 12 issues a year at a cost of $30. You can write to them at Environmental Nutrition, PO Box 420057, Palm Coast, FL 32142-9585 for more information or to subscribe.

Nutrition Action Healthletter publishes 10 issues a year at a cost of $20. This newsletter isn't shy about exposing bad food manufacturers and unhealthy eateries. It is produced by the Center for Science in the Public Interest (CSPI). Write to them at 1875 Connecticut Avenue, N.W. Suite 300. Washington, DC 20009 for more information or to subscribe.

Green Guide is a monthly newsletter that provides accurate information about health and environmental concerns. They advise about products with high levels of chemicals and how to make your own cleansers from inexpensive and nontoxic household ingredients. The publish six issues a year at a cost of $10. Write to them at Prince Street Station, PO Box 567, New York, NY 10012.

EatingWell, the Magazine of Food & Health is very visually appealing. This magazine is part health newsletter and part recipes and great food photos. *EatingWell* publishes four issues a year at a cost of $16.97. Write to them at this address: EatingWell, 823A Ferry Road, Charlotte, VT 05445. Check them out online at www.eatingwell.com.

I hope this book has helped make this time in your life a little easier—if so, my mission has been accomplished. Please write and share your stories. All best wishes for a healthy mom and a healthy baby!

Miriam Erick, MS, RD
c/o Bull Publishing Co.
P.O. Box 1377
Boulder, CO 80306

Bibliography

Accetta SG, Abeche AM, Buchabqui JA, Hames L, Pratti R, Afler T, Capp E. Memory loss and ataxia after hyperemesis gravidarum: a case of Wernicke's encephalopathy. *Eur J Ob Gyn Repro Biol.* 2002;102:100–101.

Alfaro-LeFevre R, Blicharz ME, Flynn NM, Boyer MJ. *Drug Handbook: A Nursing Process Approach.* Reading, Mass: Addison-Wesley; 1992.

Armstrong L. Weather Patterns and Air Ions. In: *Performing in Extreme Environments.* Champaign, IL: Human Kinetics. 2000:237–249.

Bart JL, Bouque DA. Acknowledging the weather-health link. *CMAJ.* Oct 1995; 153(7):941–944.

Bensoussan A. *The Vital Meridian: A Modern Exploration of Acupuncture.* New York, NY: Churchill Livingstone; 1991: 26, 34, 90–92.

Bensoussan A, Myers SP, Carlton AL. Risks associated with the practice of Traditional Chinese Medicine. *Arch Fam Med.* 2000;9:1071–1078.

Bergin PS, Harvey P. Wernicke's encephalopathy and central pontine myelinolysis associated with hyperemesis gravidarum. *Br J Med.* 1992;305:517–518.

Blass JP, Gibson GE. Abnormality of a thiamine-requiring enzyme in patients with Wernicke's encephalopathy. NEJM. 1970;297(25):1367–1370.

Bloch AS, Mueller C. Enteral and parenteral nutrition support. In: Mahan LK and Escott-Stump S, eds. Krause's Food, Nutrition, and Diet Therapy. 10th ed. Philadelphia, Penn: W.B. Saunders Co; 2000:463–482.

Borison HL, Borison R, McCarthy LE. Phylogenic and neurologic aspects of the vomiting process. J Clin Pharmacol. 1981;21:23S–29S.

Borowski KS, et al. The impact of hyperemesis gravidarum on pregnancy outcome. Obstet Gynecol. April 2003;101(4S):86S.

Bourgeois JA, et al. Clinical manifestations and management of conversion disorder. Curr Treat Options Neurol. Nov 2002;4(6):487–497.

Bourne JG. Apache Medicine-Men. New York, NY: Dover Publications; 1993.

Bowers N. The Multiple Pregnancy Sourcebook: Pregnancy and the First Days with Twins, Triplets, and More. New York, NY: McGraw Hill/ Contemporary Books; 2001.

Brizova J. The Czechoslovak Cookbook. The Crown Classic Cookbook Series. New York, NY: Crown Publishers; 1965.

Brooke E. Women Healers through History. London: Women's Press. London; 1993.

Burmucicu R, Weiss RA. Hyperemesis gravidarum and excretion of chorionic gonadotropin in collected 24-hour urine. [in German]. Geburtshilfe Frauenheildk. Feb 1987;47(2):111–112.

Byrne BM, Stronge JM. Wernicke's encephalopathy presenting in the puerperium. Ir Med J. Jul-Aug 1996;89(4):145–146.

Carlsson CPO, Axemo P, Bodin A, Carstensen H, Ehrenroth B, Madegard-Lind I, Navander C. Manual acupuncture reduces hyperemesis gravidarum: a placebo-controlled randomized, single-blind, crossover study. J Pain Symptom Manage. 2000;20(4):273–279.

Carroll C. Hyperemesis gravidarum. In: Rivlin ME, Morrison JC, Bates GW, eds. Manual of Clinical Problems in Obstetrics and Gynecology. 2nd ed. Boston, Mass: Little, Brown; 1986.

Cedard L, Guichard A, Janssen Y, Tanguy G, Boyer P, Zorn RF. Progesterone and estradiol in saliva after in vitro infertilization and embryo transfer. *Fertil Steril*. Feb 1987;47(2):278–283.

Champion T. Personal communication. 8/7/2003. Canaries in the Mines.

Chang GY. Acute Wernicke's syndrome mimicking brainstem stroke. *Eur Neurol*. 2000;43(4):246–247.

Changxin Z. Acupuncture treatment of morning sickness. *J Trad Chin Med*. 1988;8(3):228–229.

Chaturachinda K, McGregor EM. Wernicke's encephalopathy and pregnancy. *J Obst Gynec Brit Cwlth*. Sept 1968;75:969–971.

Chatwani A, Schwartz R. A severe case of hyperemesis gravidarum. *AJOG*. 1982;143(8):964–965.

Cherney, JV. *Acupuncture without Needles*. New York, NY: Penguin Putnam; 1999.

Chirino O, Kavac R, Bale D, Blythe JG. Barogenic rupture of the esophagus associated with hyperemesis gravidarum. *Obstet Gynecol*. 1978:52S:51S–53S.

Classen C, Howes D, Synnett A. *Aroma: A Cultural History of Smell*. New York, NY: Routledge. 1994.

Colucci WS, Gimbrone MA, McLaughlin MK, Halpern W, Alexander RW. Increases vascular catecholamine sensitivity and a-adrenergic receptor affininity in female and estrogen-treated male rats. *Circ Res*. 1982;50:805–811.

Combs GF. Vitamins. In: Mahan LK, Escott-Stump S, eds. *Krause's Food, Nutrition, and Diet Therapy*. 10th ed. Philadelphia, Penn: WB Saunders; 2000. 67–109.

Cook CCH, Tomson AD. B-Complex vitamins in the prophylaxis and treatment of Wernicke-Korsakoff syndrome. *Br J Hosp Med*. 1997; 57(9):461–465.

Corcoran DW, Houston T. Is the lemon test an index of arousal level? *Br J Psych*. Aug 1977;68(3):361–364.

Corcoran DWJ, Hujduk J. What does the lemon test measure? *Biol Psych.* 1980;10:277–281.

Cordes L. *The Reflecting Pond: Meditations for Self-Discovery.* New York, NY: Harper and Row; 1986.

Coronios-Vargus M, et al. Cultural influences on food cravings and aversions during pregnancy. *Ecology of Food and Nutrition.* United Kingdom. 25(Paper 1050):1–6

Cowley DR, Dager SR, McClellan J, Roy-Byrne PP, Dunner DL. Response to lactate infusion in generalized anxiety disorder. *Biol Psychiatry.* Aug 1988;24(4):409–414.

Dager SR, Rainey JM, Kenny MA, Artru AA, Metzger GD, Bowden DM. Central nervous system effects of lactate infusion in primates. *Biol Psychiatry.* Jan 15, 1990;27(2):193–204.

Dastur FN. A controlled longitudinal study of olfactory perception and symptoms of pregnancy sickness. PhD dissertation, Dalhousie University, Halifax, Nova Scotia. May 2000.

David ML, Doyle EW. First trimester pregnancy. *Am J Nursing.* Dec 1976:1945–1948.

Davis B, Melina V. *Becoming Vegan: The Complete Guide to Adopting a Healthy Plant-Based Diet.* Summertown, Tenn: Book Publishing Company; 2000.

Davis CJ, Lake-Bakaar GV, Grahame-Smith DG, eds. *Nausea and Vomiting: Mechanisms and Treatment.* New York, NY: Springer-Verlag; 1984.

De Aloysio D, Penacchioni P. Morning sickness control in early pregnancy by neiguan point acupressure. *Obstet Gynecol.* 1992;80:852–854.

de Mar Melero-Montes M, Jick H. Hyperemesis gravidarum and the sex of the offspring. *Epidemiology.* Jan 2000;12(1):123–124.

Den Boer JA, Westenberg HG, Klompmakers AA, van Lint LE. Behavioral biochemical and neuroendocrine concomitants of lactate-induced panic anxiety. *Biol Psychiatry.* Oct 1989;26(6):612–622.

DePue RH, et al. Hyperemesis gravidarum in relation to estradiol levels, pregnancy outcome, and other maternal factors: a seroepidemiologic study. *Am J Obstet Gynecol.* 1987;156:1137–1141.

Deuelle P, et al. Hyperemesis in the first trimester of pregnancy: role of biological hyperthyroidism and fetal sex. *Gynecol Obstet Fertil.* Mar 2002;30(3):204–209.

Diav-Citrin O, Koren G. Human Teratogens. In: Koren G, Bishai R, eds. *Nausea and Vomiting of Pregnancy: State of the Art 2000.* Motherisk, the Hospital for Sick Children. Toronto, Canada. 181–193.

Dossey L. *Healing Words: The Power of Prayer and the Practice of Medicine.* San Francisco, CA: HarperSanFrancisco; 1993.

Drevelengas A, Chourmouzi D, Pitsavas G, Charitandi A, Boulogianni G. Reversible brain atrophy and subcortical high signal on MRI in a patient with anorexia nervosa. *Neuroradiology.* 2001;43:838–840.

Duke JA. *Handbook of Northeastern Indian Medicinal Plants.* Lawrence, Mass: Quarterman Publications; 1986.

Eddy MB. *Science and Health with Key to the Scriptures.* Boston: First Church of Christ, Scientist; 1911.

El-Mallakh RS, Liebowitz RN, Hale MS. Hyperemesis gravidarum as conversion disorder. *J Ner Mental Ds.* 1990;178(10):655–659.

Environmental Nutrition (the newsletter of food, nutrition, and health). What can you do to lick a chronic dry mouth problem? Jan 2004;27(1):7.

Ergil KV. Acupuncture licensure, training, and certification in the United States. In: "NIH Consensus Development Conference on Acupuncture." Office of Alternative Medicine, Office of Medical Applications of Research. Bethesda, MD. Proceedings of the conference. November 3–5, 1997: 31–38.

Erichsen-Brown C. *Medicinal and Other Uses of North American Plants: A Historical Survey with Special Reference to the Eastern Indian Tribes.* New York, NY: Dover Publications; 1979.

Erick M. Hyperemesis gravidarum: a practical management strategy. *OBG Management*. 2000;12(11):25–28, 33–35.

Erick M. Hyperemesis gravidarum and morning sickness: insights from sufferers and medical literature. Panel discussion presented at Food and Nutrition Conference and Exhibition. American Dietetic Association. San Antonio, Tex; October 26, 2003.

Erick M. Hyperolfaction and hyperemesis gravidarum: what is the relationship? *Nutr Rev*. Oct 1995;53(10):289–295.

Erick M. Malnutrition Awareness Activity. *J Am Diet Assoc*. Sept 2000;100(9):1004–1006.

Erick M. Morning sickness impact study. *Midwifery Today*. Autumn 2001; 59:30–32.

Erick M. Ptylism gravidarum: an unpleasant reality. *J Am Diet Assoc*. 1998;98(2):129.

Erick M. *Take Two Crackers and Call Me in the Morning! A Real-Life Guide for Surviving Morning Sickness*. Brookline, Mass: Grinnen-Barrett Publishing Company; 1995.

Erick M, Bunnell MK. Nausea and vomiting of pregnancy: manifestations and current intervention. *Female Patient*. Oct 2000; 25(10):59–69.

Fairweather DVI. Nausea and vomiting in pregnancy. *American Journal of Ob Gyn*. Sept 1, 1968;102(1):135–175.

Fait V, et al. Hyperemesis gravidarum is associated with oxidative stress. *Am J Perinat*. 2002:19(2):93–98.

Flannelly G, Turner JM, Connolly R, Stronge JM. Persistent hyperemesis gravidarum complicated by Wernicke's encephalopathy. *Irish J Med Sci*. 1990;159:82.

Flemming G. The importance of air quality in human biometeorology. *Int J Biometeorol*. Nov 1996;39(4):192–196.

Fletcher RJ. "Fohn illness" and human biometeorology in the Chinook area of Canada. *Int J Biometerol*. Sep 1988;32(3):168–75.

Folk JJ, Leslie HFM. Hyperemesis gravidarum: pregnancy outcomes and complications among women nutritionally supported with and without parenteral therapy. (Abstract for CME April-May 2001 Chicago) *Obstet Gynecol.* April 2001;97(4):42S.

Frank LE. *Native American Cooking: Foods of the Southwest Indian Nations.* New York, NY: Clarkson Potter Publishers; 1991.

Franko DL, Spurrel EB. Detection and management of eating disorders during pregnancy. *Ob Gyn.* 2000;95:942–946.

Fraser D. Central pontine myelinolysis as a result of hyperemesis gravidarum: case report. *Br J Ob Gyn.* 1988;95:621–623.

Fyer AJ, Liebowitz MR, Gorman JM, Davies SO, Klein DF. Lactate vulnerability of remitted panic patients. *Psychiatry Res.* Feb 1985;14(2):143–148.

Gardian G, Voros E, Jardanhazy T, Ungurean A, Vecsei L. Wernicke's encephalopathy induced by hyperemesis gravidarum. Case report. *Acta Neurol Scand.* 1999;99:196–198.

Gawande A. Medical Dispatch: A queasy feeling: the ups and downs of trying to treat nausea. *New Yorker.* July 15, 1999:34–41.

Gilmore MR. *Uses of Plants by the Indians of the Missouri River Region.* Lincoln: University of Nebraska Press; 1991.

Gorbach JS, Counselman FL, Mendelson MH. Spontaneous pneumomediastinum secondary to hyperemesis gravidarum. *J Emerg Med.* Sept-Oct 1997;15(5):639–643.

Groopman J. *The Anatomy of Hope: How People Prevail in the Face of Illness.* New York, NY: Random House; 2004.

Gruber HE, Gutteridge DH, Baylink DJ. Osteoporosis associated with pregnancy and lactation: bone density and skeletal features in three patients. *Metab Bone Dis Related Res.* 1984;5(4):159–165.

Guen R (dentist). Personal communication. Brookline, Mass; Oct 2003.

Hall MJ, Schappert SM. National Center for Health Statistics, Division of Health Care Statistics. Personal communication (via Internet).

Hammond, KA. Dietary and Clinical Assessment. In: Mahan and Escott-Stump, eds. *Krause's Food, Nutrition, and Diet Therapy.* 10th ed. Philadelphia: WB Saunders; 2000.

Han, J. Acupuncture actives endogenous systems of analgesia. In: "NIH Consensus Development Conference on Acupuncture." Bethesda, MD. November 3–5, 1997: 55–60.

Hardy JD. Biometeorology: physiological and behavioral perspectives. *Int J Biometeorol*. 1976;6(2 Suppl):29–35.

Harris JB. *Iron Pots and Wooden Spoons: 175 Authentic Cajun, Creole and Caribbean Dishes*. New York, NY: Ballantine Books; 1989.

Hart AD. *Dark Clouds, Silver Linings*. Colorado Springs, Colo: Focus on the Family Publishing; 1993.

Hasse JM, Matarese LE. Medical nutrition therapy for liver, biliary system, and exocrine pancreas disorders. In: Mahan LK and Escott-Stump S, eds. *Krause's Food, Nutrition, and Diet Therapy*. 10th ed. Philadelphia: WB Saunders; 2000:695–721.

Haynes C. *2,002 Ways to Cheer Yourself Up*. Kansas City, Mo: Andrews McMeel Publishing; 1998.

Heinrichs WL. Linking olfaction with nausea and vomiting of pregnancy, recurrent abortion, hyperemesis gravidarum, and migraine headaches. *Headache*. Mar 2003;43(3):304–305.

Hendrie R (compiled by). *Ouma's Cookery Book*. Capetown, South Africa: Juta & Co.; 1940.

Henry RJW, Vadas RA. Spontaneous rupture of the oesophagus following severe vomiting in early pregnancy. Case report. *Br J Ob Gyn*. 1986;93:392–394.

Hill JB, Yost NP, Wendel GD. Acute renal failure in association with hyperemesis gravidarum. *Obstet Gynecol*. 2002;100:1119–1121

Hill JM. *Practical Cooking and Serving*. New York: Doubleday, Page & Co.; 1921.

Hillbom M, Pyhtinen J, Pylvanen V, Sotaniemi K. Pregnant, vomiting, and coma. *Lancet*. May 8, 1999;353:1584.

Hoffer LJ. Starvation. In: Shils ME, Young VR, eds. *Modern Nutrition in Health and Disease*. 7th ed.. Philadephia, Penn:Lea & Febiger. 1988:774–794.

Holt V, Cushing-Haugen KL, Daling JR. Oral contraceptives, tubal sterilization, and functional ovarian cyst risk. *Obstet Gynecol.* Aug 2003;102(2):252–258.

Hoppe P. Aspects of human biometeorology in past, present, and future. *Int J Biometerol.* Feb 1997;40(1):19–23

Huddleston P. *Prepare for Surgery, Heal Faster.* Cambridge, Mass: Angel River Press; 1996.

Hughes WL, Robinson AC. Treatment of hyperemesis gravidarum with intramuscular injections of husband's blood. *Am J Ob Gyn.* July-Dec 1942;(44):103–105.

Hultman T, ed. *The African News Cookbook: African Cooking for Western Kitchens.* Middlesex, England: Penguin Books; 1985.

Hutchens AR. *Indian Herbalogy of North America.* Boston, Mass: Shambhala; 1973.

Info to go. Getting enough of a good thing: fructooligosaccharies (FOS). *J Am Diet Assoc.* Nov 1988:534.

Jarnfelt-Samsioe A, et al. Gallbladder disease related to the use of oral contraceptives and nausea in pregnancy. *S Med J.* Sept 1985;78(9):1040–1043.

Jarnfelt-Samsioe A, Bremme K, Eneroth P. Non-steroid hormones and tissue polypeptide antigen in emetic and non-emetic pregnancies. *Acta Obstet Gynecol Scand.* 1986;65:745–751.

Jarnsfelt-Samsioe A, Samsioe G, Velinger Gun-Marie. Nausea and vomiting in pregnancy—a contribution to its epidemiology. *Gynecol Obstet Invest.* 1983;16:221–229.

Jednak, MA et al. Protein meals reduce nausea and gastric slow wave dysrhythmic activity in first trimester pregnancy. *Am J Physiol.* 1999;40:G855–G861.

Kaledin E. *The Morning Sickness Companion.* New York, NY: St. Martins Press; 2003.

Kanayama N, Khatun S, Belayet HM, Yamashita M, Yonezawa M, Kobayashi T. Terao T. Vasospasms of cerebral arteries in hyperemesis gravidarum. *Gyn Obst Invest*. Aug 1998;46(2):139–141.

Kanosue K, Matsuo R, Tanaka H. Nakayama T. Effect of body temperature on salivary reflexes in rats. *J Auton Nerve Syst*. July 1986;15(3):233–237.

Kavasch B. *Native Harvests*. New York, NY: Vintage Books. 1979.

Kavasch EB. *Enduring Harvests: Native American Foods and Festivals for Every Season*. Old Saybrook, Conn: Globe Pequot Press; 1995.

Kawakami Sho-Ichi, et al. Effect of Chinese herbal medicine suppositories for hyperemsis gravidarum by using an index for nausea and vomiting of pregnancy. In: Koren G, Bishai R, eds. *Nausea and Vomiting of Pregnancy: State of the Art 2000*. Motherisk, the Hospital for Sick Children. Toronto, Canada; 2000: 122–127.

Kemp WN. Hyperemesis gravidarum treated as a temporary adrenal cortex insufficiency. *Lancet*. April 1933:389–391.

Kim Y, Lee S, Rah S, Lee J. Wernicke's encephalopathy in hyperemesis gravidarum. *Can J Opthal*. 2002;37:37–38.

Klebanoff M, et al. Epidemiology of vomiting in early pregnancy. *Ob Gyn*. 1985;66(5):612–661.

Klein BT. *Reference Encyclopedia of the American Indian*. 6th ed. West Nyack, NY: Todd Publications 1993.

Knight B, Mudge C, Openshaw S, White A, Hart A. Effect of Acupuncture on nausea of pregnancy: a randomized, controlled trial. *Ob Gyn*. 2001;97:184–188.

Koch KL, Stern RM, Vasey M, Botti GW, Creasy GW, Dwyer A. Gastric dysrthythmias and nausea of pregnancy. *Dig Dig Sc*. Aug 1990;35(8):961–968.

Kohlmeir LA, Federman M, Leboff MS. Osteomalacia and osteoporosis in a woman with anklyosing spondylitis. *J Bone Min Res*. 1996;11(5):697–703.

Krzywicki HJ, Consolazio CF, Matoush LO, Johnson HL. Metabolic aspects of acute starvation. *A J Clin Nutr*. 1968;1(21):87–97.

Lavin PJM, Smith D, Kori SH, Ellenberger C. Wernicke's encephalopathy: a predictable complication of hyperemesis gravidarum. *Obstet Gynecol.* 1983;62:13S.

Lee TA, et al. Compositional changes in brewed coffee as a function of brewing time. *Journal of Food Science.* 1992;57(6):1417–1419.

LeGuerer A. *Scent: The Mysterious and Essential Powers of Smell.* Turtle Bay Books, a division of Random House. 1992.

Leung AL. *Chinese Herbal Remedies.* Universe Books. 1984.

Lewis JS. Symptoms of pregnancy in fathers-to-be. *New York Times.* April 3, 1985; Section C12.

Lian YL, Chen CY, Hammes M, Kolster BC. *The Seirin Pictorial Atlas of Acupuncture: An Illustrated Manual of Acupuncture Points.* Ogal HP, Stor W, eds. Marburg, Germany: KMV-Verlag; 1999: 15.

Lipkin M, Lamb GS. The Couvade syndrome: an epidemiologic study. *Annals of Internal Medicine.* 1982;96:509–511.

Locke-Doone N. *Indian Doctor.* Charlotte, NC: Aerial Photography Services, Inc. 1985.

Longfelder, Tinker, Kidman, Attorneys at Law. Personal communication. Seattle, Washington; 1999.

Lorris BA, Goldstein GW, Katzman R. Blood-brain cerebrospinal fluid barriers. In: Siegel G, Agranoff B, Albers RW, Molinoff P, eds. *Basic Neurochemistry.* 4th ed. New York, NY: Raven Press; 1989. 591–606.

Lu HC. *Chinese System of Food Cures: Prevention and Remedies.* New York, NY: Sterling Publishing; 1986.

Maddock RJ, Mateo-Bermudez J. Elevated serum lactate following hyperventilation during glucose infusion in panic disorder. *Biol Psychiatry.* Feb 15,1990;27(4):411–418.

Maloni JA, et al. Physical and psychological side effects of ante partum hospital bed rest. *Nursing Research.* July-Aug 1993;42(4):197–203.

Marks C, Soeharjo M. *The Indonesian Kitchen.* New York, NY: Atheneum Books. 1981.

Masson JM. The Nine Emotional Lives of Cats: A Journey into the Feline Heart. New York, NY: Ballantine Books; 2002. 72.

Maternal iron deficiency affects carnitine metabolism in rat pups. Nutr Rev. 1985;43(7):220–222.

Mayat Z. Indian Delights: A Book on Indian Cookery. Durban, South Africa: Women's Cultural Group; 1961.

Mazzotta P, et al. Attitudes, management, and consequences of nausea and vomiting of pregnancy in the United States and Canada. Intl Jour Gyn Obstet. 2000;70:359–365.

Mazzota P, Magee L, Koren G. Therapeutic abortion due to severe morning sickness: unacceptable combination. Canadian Fam Phys. June 1997:1055–1057.

McIntyre A. The Medicinal Garden: How to Grow and Use Your Own Medicinal Herbs. New York, NY: Owl Books. 1997.

McLean J. Wernicke's encephalopathy induced by magnesium deficiency. Lancet. May 22, 1999;353:1768.

Merchant I. Ismail Merchant's Indian Cuisine. New York, NY: Fireside Books; 1986.

Milea D, et al. Blindness in a vegan. NEJM. Mar 23, 2000;342(12):897–898.

Moore M. Los Remedies de la Gente: A complilation of Traditional New Mexican Herbal Medicines and Their Uses. (A booklet) Santa Fe, NM 1977.

Moore M. Medicinal Plants of the Desert and Canyon West. Santa Fe, NM: Museum of New Mexico Press; 1989.

Moore M. Medicinal Plants of the Pacific West. Santa Fe, NM: Red Crane Books; 1993.

Moran P, Taylor R. Management of hyperemesis gravidarum: the importance of weight loss as a criterion for steroid therapy. QJ Med. 2002;95:153–158.

Morgane PJ, Austin-LaFrance RJ, Bronzino JD, Tonkiss J, Galler JR. Malnutrition and the developing nervous system. In: Isaacson RL,

Jensen KF, eds. *The Vulnerable Brain and Environmental Risks*, vol. 1. New York, NY: Plenum: 1992. 3–43.

Morita M, Takeda N, Hasegawa S, Yamatodani A, Wada, H, Sakai, S, Kubo T, Matsunaga T. Effects of anticholinergic and cholinergic drugs on habituation to motion in rats. [in Swedish]. *Acta Otolaryngol.* 1990;110:196–202.

Morris S. *Southeast Asian Cookery: An Authenic Taste of the Orient.* London: Grafton Books; 1989.

Moskowitz R. *Homeopathic Medicines for Pregnancy and Childbirth.* Berkeley, Calif: North Atlantic Books. 1992.

Munch S. A qualitative analysis of physician humanism: women's experiences with hyperemesis gravidarum. *J Perinatology.* 2000;20:540–547.

Munch S. Chicken or the egg? The biological-psychological controversy surrounding hyperemesis gravidarum. *Soc Sci Med.* 2002;55:1267–1278.

Munch S. Personal communication, 8/7/2003.

Munch S. Women's experiences with a pregnancy complication: causal explanations of hyperemesis gravidarum. *Social Work in Health Care.* 2002;36(1):59–75.

Munsen S. *Cooking the Norwegian Way.* Minneapolis, MN: Lerner Publications; 1982.

Murphey E. *Indian Uses of Native Plants.* Glenwood, Ill: Meyerbooks; 1990.

Murphy GT. Human chorionic gonadotropin and hyperemesis gravidarum. In: Koren G, Bishai R, eds. *Nausea and Vomiting of Pregnancy: State of the Art 2000.* Toronto: Motherisk Program; 1999:15–22.

Ngo B, Zimmerman G. *The Classic Cuisine of Vietnam.* New York, NY: Plume; 1986.

Ngugen N, Deitel M, Lacy E. Splenic avulsion in a pregnant patient with vomiting. *Can J Surg.* 1995;38(5):464–465.

Nichot P, Guichard JP, Djomby R, Sellier P, Bousser MG, Chabriat H. Transient decrease of water diffusion in Wernicke's encephalopathy. *Neuroradiology.* 2002;44:305–307.

Nightingale S, Bates D, Heath PD, Barron SL. Wernicke's encephalopathy in hyperemesis gravidarum. *Postgrad Med J.* Sept 1982;58:558–559.

"NIH Consensus Development Conference on Acupuncture." Bethesda, MD: Office of Alternative Medicine, Office of Medical Applications of Research. November 3–5, 1997.

O'Connor S. *The Irish Isle.* Emeryville, CA: Menus and Music Productions; 1997.

Ogershok PR, Rahman A, Nestor S. Wernicke's encephalopathy in nonalcoholic patients. *Am J Med Sci.* 2002;323(2):107–111.

Ohkoshi N, Ishii A, Shoji S. Wernicke's encephalopathy induced by hyperemesis gravidarum, associated with bilateral caudate lesions on computed tomography and magnetic resonance imaging. *Eur Neurol.* 1994;34:177–180.

Omer SM, al Kawi MZ, al Watban J, Bohlega S, McLean DR, Miller G. Acute Wernicke's encephalopathy associated with hyperemesis gravidarum: magnetic resonance imaging findings. *J Neuroimagining.* Oct 1995;5(4):251–253.

Orji EO, Ogunlol IO, Fasubaa OB. Sexuality among pregnant women in southwest Nigeria. *J Ob Gyn.* Mar 2002;22(2):166–168.

Ortiz EL. *The Book of Latin American Cooking.* New York, NY: Penguin Books; 1985.

Ortiz EL. *The Complete Book of Caribbean Cooking.* New York, NY: Ballantine Books; 1973.

Ovsiew F. What is wrong in conversion disorder? *J Neurol Neurosurg Psychiatry.* May 2003;74(5):557.

Oxenford R. *Instant Reflexology or Stress Relief: Simple Techniques to Relieve Stress and Enhance Your Mind.* New York, NY: Barnes and Noble Books; 2002.

Pantoflickova D, et. al. Favourable effect of regular intake of fermented milk containing Lactobaililus johnsonii on Helicobacter pylori associated gastritis. *Aliment Pharmacol Ther.* Oct 15, 2003; 18(8):805–813.

Parfitt A. Nausea and vomiting. In: "NIH Consensus Development Conference on Acupuncture." Bethesda, MD. November 3–5, 1997: 91.

Parsons, EC, ed. *North American Indian Life.* New York, NY: Dover Publications; 1992.

Peeters A, Van De Wyngaert F, Van Lierde M, Sindic CJM, Laterre EC. Wernicke's encephalopathy and central pontine myelinolysis induced by hyperemesis gravidarum. *Acta neurolg belg.* 1993;93:276–282.

Persinger MA. Mental process and disorders: a neurobehavioral perspective in human biometeorology. *Experientia.* Jan 15, 1987;43(1):39–48.

Petusevsky S, et al. *The Whole Foods Market Cookbook: A Guide to Natural Foods with 350 Recipes.* New York, NY: Clarkson Potter Publishers; 2002.

Postolache T. Psychopharmacology Consultation Service, St. Elizabeth's Hospital, District of Columbia. Department of Mental Health, Washington, D.C. National Institute of Mental Health and Department of Psychiatry, University of Maryland, Baltimore. Personal communication. Lemons, depression, mood, and seasonal-affective disorder. Sept 8, 2003.

Pregnant? Say No to Soy. *Prevention Magazine.* Sept 2003:60.

Profet M. *Protecting Your Baby-to-Be.* Reading, MA: Addison Wesley 1995.

Rees JH, Ginsberg L, Schapira AHV. Two pregnant women with vomiting and fits. *Am J Obstet Gynecol.* 1997;177:1539–1540.

Robinson D, Casso DE, Omar SJ, Tinklenberg JR. Possible oral lactate exacerbation of panic attack. *Annals of Pharmacotherapy.* May 1995;29:539–540.

Robinson JN, Banerjee R, Thiet MP. Coagulopathy secondary to vitamin K deficiency in hyperemesis gravidarum. *Ob Gyn.* Oct 1998;92(4 pt 2):673–675.

Rogers PJ, Hill AJ. Breakdown of dietary restraint following mere exposure to food stimuli: interrelationship between restrict, hunger, salivation and food intake. *Addict Behav.* 1989;14(4):387–397.

Romo I. *Homestyle Mexican Cooking.* Chicago, Ill: Surrey Books; 1988.

Rongun Z. Thirty-nine cases of morning sickness treated with acupuncture. *J Trad Chin Med.* 1987;7(1):25–26.

Rose RS. *Feeding the Family.* New York, NY: MacMillian Co.; 1917.

Rotman P, Hassin D, Mouallem, Barkai G, Farfel Z. Wernicke's encephalopathy in hyperemesis gravidarum with abnormal liver function. *Isr J Med Sci.* 1994;30:225–228.

Salonen V, Nikoskelanine J, Heinonen OJ, Kalimo H. Aula P. Carnitine deficiency and severe nausea-induced thiamine deficiency causing a metabolic crisis [in Finnish]. *Duodecim.* 1992;108(11):1059–1062.

Schiffman S. Taste and smell in disease. *NEJM.* May 26, 1983;308(21):1275–1279.

Schuh A. Climatotherapy. *Experientia.* Nov 15, 1993;49(11):947–956.

Schuler E. *German Cookery.* The Crown Cookbook Series. New York, NY: Crown Publishers; 1983.

Schwartz M, Rossoff L. Pneumonmediastinum and bilateral pneumothraces in a patient with hyperemesis gravidarum. *Chest.* 1994;106:1904–1906.

Scialli AR. Burden of disease. Nausea and vomiting of pregnancy: What's new? Conference proceedings. The Reproductive Toxicology Center. Washington, D.C. Sept 2000.

Sechi G, Serra A, Pirastru MI, Sotgiu S, Rosati G. Wernicke's encephalopathy in a woman on a slimming diet. *Neurology.* Jun 11, 2002;58(11):1697–1698.

Seely C, ed. *Ginger Up Your Cookery.* London: Hutchinson Benham; 1977.

Serfini M, et al. Total antioxidant potential of fruit and vegetables and risk of gastric cancer. *Gastroenterology.* Oct 2002; 123(4):985–991.

Sibilia J, Javier RM, Werle C, Kuntz JL. Fracture of the sacrum in the absence of osteoporosis of pregnancy: a rare skeletal complication of the postpartum. *Br J Ob Gyn.* Oct 1999;106:1096–1097.

Signorello LB, Harlow BL, Wang S, Erick MA. Saturated fat intake and the risk of severe hyperemesis gravidarum. *Epidemiology.* Nov 1998;9(6):636–640.

Simon EP, Schwartz J. Medical hypnosis for hyperemesis gravidarum. *Birth.* Dec 1999; 26:4:248–254.

Simopoulos AP, Robinson J. *The Omega Diet The Life-Saving Nutritional Program Based on the Diet of the Island of Crete.* New York, NY: Harper Perennial; 1999.

Skoura S. *The Greek Cookbook.* The Crown Classic Cookbook Series. New York, NY: Crown Publishers; 1967.

Smith RA, Nelson CS. Oesophageal obstruction following hyperemesis gravidarum. *Thorax.* 1965;20:528–531.

Sokoloff L. Circulation and energy metabolism of the brain. In: Seigel G, Agranoff B, Albers RW, Molinoff P, eds. *Basic Neurochemistry.* 4th ed. New York, NY: Raven Press; 1989:565–590.

Somer E. *Nutrition for a Healthy Pregnancy: The Complete Guide to Eating Before, During, or After Your Pregnancy.* Rev ed. New York, NY: Owl Books; 2002.

Spruill SC, Kuller JA. Hyperemesis gravidarum complicated by Wernicke's encphalopathy. *Obstet Gynecol.* 2002;99:875–877.

Stevenson MC. *The Zuni Indians and Their Use of Plants.* New York, NY: Dover Publications; 1993.

Stoll AL. *The Omega 3 Connection.* New York, NY: Simon and Schuster; 2001.

Sufi SB, Donaldson A, Gandy SC, Jeffcoate SL, Chearskul S, Goh H, Hazra D, Romero C, Wang HZ. Multicenter evaluation of assays for estradiol and progesterone in saliva. *Clin Chem.* Jan 1985; 31(1):101–103.

Tan LT, Tan MYC, Veith I. *Acupuncture Therapy: Current Chinese Practice.* 2nd ed. (revised and enlarged). Philadelphia, PA: Temple University Press; 1976: 26, 205.

Tesfaye S, Achari V, Chenu Yang Y, Harding S, Bowden A, Yora JP. Pregnant, vomiting, and going blind. *Lancet.* Nov 14, 1998:1594.

Tierson F, Olsen C, Hook E. Nausea and vomiting of pregnancy and association with pregnancy outcome. *AJOG.* 1986:1017–1022.

Togay-Isikay C, Yigit A, Mutluer N. Wernicke's encephalopathy due to hyperemesis gravidarum: an under-recognised condition. *Aust NZ Obstet Gynaecol Suppl.* Nov 2001; 41(4):453–456.

Train P, Henrichs JR, Archer WA. *Medicinal Uses of Plants by Indian Tribes of Nevada.* Lawrence, Mass: Quarterman Publications; 1957.

Tsay, KS. *Acupuncturist's Handbook: A Practical Encyclopedia.* 3rd ed. Newton Centre, MA: CPM Whole Health; 2000.

Tylden E. Hyperemesis and physiological vomiting. *J Psychsomatic Research.* 1968;(12):85–93.

Van Dinter MC. Ptyalism in Pregnancy. In: *Women and Reproductive Nutrition Report.* (newsletter of the Women and Reproductive Nutrition Dietetic Practice Group of the American Dietetic Association). Fall 2002;4(1):1–4.

van Wyk M. *Cooking the South African Way.* Johannesburg, South Africa: Central News Agency; 1986.

Venter EK, et al. Conversion disorder and calcium homeostatis. *S Afr Med J.* Dec 2002;92(12):970–971.

Vomiting of Pregnancy: A Symposium of the Current Literature. New Haven, Conn.: BiSoDol Company; 1932

Wagner S and Breiteneder H. The latex-fruit syndrome. Biochemical Society Meeting: Plant Food Allergens: Industrial Biochemistry and Biotechnology Group. July, 18, 2002; 935–940.

Wakui W, Nishimura S, Watahibi Y, Endo Y, Nakamoto Y, Miura AB. Dramatic recovery from neurological deficits in a patient with central pontine myelinolysis following severe hyponatremia. *Jpn J Med.* May-June 1991;30(3):281–284.

Walker ARP, Walker BF, Jones J, Veradi M, Walker C. Nausea and vomiting and dietary cravings and aversions during pregancy in South African women. *Br J Obstet Gynecol.* 1985;92:484–489.

Wallace LH. *The Rumford Complete Cookbook.* Rumford, RI: Rumford Company; 1931.

Walters WAW. The management of nausea and vomiting in pregnancy. *Med Jour Austral.* Sept 21, 1987;147:290–291.

Wantanabe K, Tanaka K, Masuda J. Wernicke's encephalopathy in early pregnancy complicated by diseminated intravascular coagulation. *Virchows Arch A Pathol Anat Hisopathol.* 1983;400(2):213–218.

Wei-P'ing W. *Chinese Acupuncture.* (Translated and adapted by Philip M. Chancellor). Elmford, NY: British Book Centre; 1962: 139, 148.

Weiss G. The death of Charlotte Bronte. *Ob Gyn.* 1991;78(4):705–708.

West K. *The Best of Polish Cooking.* New York, NY: Weathervane Books; 1983.

Wilson LG. *The Couvade Syndrome.* 1977.

Winter R. *The Smell Book.* Philadelphia, Penn: JB Lippincott; 1976.

Wood P, Murray A, Sinha B, Goldsmith HJ. Wernicke's encephalopathy induced by hyperemesis gravidarum. Case report. *B J Ob Gyn.* 1983;90:583–586.

Woolford TJ, Birzgalis AR, Lundell C, Farrington WT. Vomiting in pregnancy resulting in oesophageal perforation in a 15-year-old. *J Largyngol Otolog.* Nov 1993; 107:1059–1060.

Yamada E. A study of the etiology of "Tsuwari" (emesis gravidarum) with a special reference to fluctuations of urinary 17 KS fractions in pregnant women with Tsuwari. [in Japanese]. *Tokyo Ika Daigaku Zasshi.* Mar 1970;28(2):155–224.

Yamaga A, Taga, M, Takahashi T, Shirai T. A case of postpregnancy osteoporosis. *E Jour Ob Gyn Repro Biol.* 2000;88:107–109.

Yoneda T, Tagashire S, Kita A, Matsurra M, Takatsuga K. A case of Wernicke's encephalopathy caused by an extremely unbalanced diet [in Japanese]. *Sangyo Eiseigaku Zasshi.* Mar 1999;41(2)21–3.

Yoneyama Y, et al. The T-helper1/T-helper 2 balance in peripheral blood of women with hyperemesis gravidarum. AJOG. Dec 2002;187:1631–1635.

Index